Chinese Feng Shui and Indian Vaastu have many things in common, but there are many varieties also which distinguish both the ancient sciences. The author has suitably and ably compared common and variable points between Feng Shui and Vaastu. So, the readers will have a first hand knowledge of both.

This is the first book of its kind on the subject which has been made useful by explaining the technical terms in English. Hopefully, this book will enlighten all and also satiate their inquisitive urge.

FENG-SHUI

CHINESE VAASTU

Chinese Vaastu for better Living and Prosperity

FENG SHUI

CHINESE VAASTU

Chinese Vaastu for better Living and Prosperity

Vaastu Samrat, Jyotish Martand

DR BHOJRAJ DWIVEDI

M.A., Phd.

Chief Editor: *Agayata Darshan* and *Shri Chandmartand Panchang*

Joint Editor

Pt Ramesh Dwivedi

M.A. (Sanskrit)

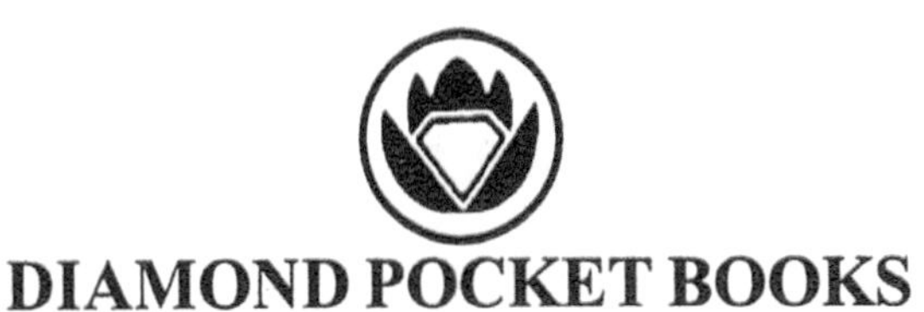

DIAMOND POCKET BOOKS

Publisher : **Diamond Pocket Books (P) Ltd.**
X-30, Okhla Industrial Area, Phase-II
New Delhi-110020
Phone : 011-40712200
E-mail : wecare@diamondbooks.in
Website : www.diamondbooks.in
Edition : 2025

FENG SHUI: CHINESE VAASTU-SHASTRA

By Dr. Bhojraj Dwivedi

Contents

Part-1
Feng Shui & Chinese Vastu Shastra

Part-2
I-Ching

Part-3
Advance Feng Shui

INTRODUCTION

There is craze for Feng Shui in India and abroad. A new word, 'Feng Shui', has appeared in many books written on Vaastu Shastra. What is implied by 'Feng Shui' and how and in what way is it related, if at all, to Vaastu Shastra? I receive so many letters daily where I have been asked many a times as to which out of the two sciences is more precise, authentic and useful.

Shri Narender Kumar, Managing Director of **Diamond Pocket Books,** has been insisting upon me to write an authentic book on Feng Shui, each in Hindi and English. Many books in foreign languages are available on the book stands but due to their high prices the aspirants are unable to purchase them. My book titled **'Feng Shui: Chinese Vaastu Shastra',** will hopefully fill in this void.

I feel privileged to present this book to the discerning readers and earnestly hope it will meet their requirements and purpose. It is due to benign kindness of Goddess Saraswati that I have been able to complete this book for the general welfare of the readers.

Which of these two sciences is more accurate and to what extent? I feel I have been provided with an opportunity to express my views in reasonable details, to explain that Feng Shui is not merely confined within the four walls of the Vaastu Shastra.

In fact, Feng Shui is a philosophy a contemplation of the ancient Chinese scholars, who have explained how natural forces impact personal life and fortune of an individual.

Ancient Chinese scholars had devised certain principles by dint of their divine experiences. They mainly dwelt upon Chinese Lunar days, Zodiac signs, annual zodiac signs, G-Ching and hexagram. These being the leading attributes of the Feng Shui and if these facets are set aside, importance and utility of Feng Shui comes to an naught. That is, we can not conceive of Feng Shui, in the absence of the said facets. This is the first authentic and reliable book wherein facts, pertaining to Feng Shui, have been authentically explained and dealt with.

Origin of Feng Shui dates back to 5000 years, and the Chinese culture is thought to be oldest culture in the world. But reference to Indian Vaastu Shastra is found in the Vedic mantras that pertain in the context of Vaastu Purush. Vedas are eternal they have neither any beginning nor an end. Till now the exact date of writing of the Vedas is unknown, but some scholars maintain that Vedas were written over twenty years. B.C.

However, much certain that Rigveda is the oldest treatise of the world. So, Feng Shui is not, at all, more ancient than the Vedic Vaastu.

In fact, Feng Shui has taken a cue from Indian Vaastu and is also influenced by the latter, and more particularly by Buddhism, which reached China via Tibet. It will not be an exaggeration if we maintain that Feng Shui's roots, along with the Chinese culture and civilization, and are embedded in Indian Vaastu Shastra and is actually a reformed version of the Indian Vaastu Shastra.

If we expand the inherent import of Feng Shui, then it denotes Chinese spiritual life style, which is based on Chinese 'Taoism'. If we wish to fully understand Feng Shui we have to deeply study the Chinese religious concept 'Tao'. If we desire to understand fully, both the Taoism and Feng Shui, we have to fully comprehend the technical terminology and its precise and apt pronunciation. So, in order to obviate readers' problems and difficulties, a glossary of important technical terms has been given at the end of the books as this aspect has been found wanting in other books written on the subject.

Almost all the principles in the Indian Vaastu Shastra and Chinese Feng Shui are identical, except, of course, that Chinese consider the South and southern direction auspicious, while in India this side is considered as ominous. The Chinese consider it auspicious to have fountains, plantations, fish houses. Water reservoirs in the south-east direction, whereas a southern door is considered as ominous in the south direction, though Chinese consider an entry gate on this side as auspicious.

Both the said principles of Feng Shui do not fit Indian Vaastru Shastra's slot, and herein lies the basic difference between the two sciences. Though notice these glaring variations are because of the climatic factors, which are totally at variance with each other.

All the rivers world over flow from North to South. The Himalayas is situated in the Northern side of India and the Ganga and the Mahanadi rivers originate from the Himalayas. The Himalayas guards the frontiers or the country on the northern side. Lord Shiva also has his seat on the top of the Himalayas, hence the northern side is auspicious for the Indians. Dead bodies are burnt in the South direction, because Lord Hanuman who had burnt Lanka, situated in the South. South direction is called a vacantsite hence it should be left open or vacant. This is the reason behind considering southern direction as an ominous or unauspicious side.

I went to Egypt during September-October 2000. Entire Egypt is dependent on the water of Nile river. Nile river is the only source of subsistence for the Egyptians and it is a boon for them. But the Nile river, unlike the Ganga flows from South to East direction, it provides greenery to six countries-this might be the reason why south was described as an auspicious direction in some of the Western countries. So, Vaastu of each region is dependant on its climate and that is why variable measuring stick are applied by each country in relation to Vaastu. Hence, an expert scholar should keep all the said factors in mind.

Wind blow in the eastern and northern directions in India and it has a salutary impact on the people, and this is why most of the doors and windows are kept in the east or north direction.

Climate in China is at total variance with that of India. Mangolia territory to the North of China, where yellow or red coloured dust winds blow, this is the reason why Chinese abstain from keeping doors and windows on the northern side because, if windows and doors are kept on the northern side, all the harmful sand and dust particles will flow into the house. So they generally keep the north-east side closed and consider southern direction auspicious. When we study Chinese science of Vaastu, we must not overlook changed geographical and climatic conditions existing in that country.

No doubt when we study Feng Shui we not only add to our knowledge but also get conversant with multifaceted and multi-coloured knowledge of this great science. Until now there was no authentic book available on the subject, and I feel my book will suitably fill up the void in this respect. But, to what extent I have been successful in my efforts, can only be decided and determined by the reaction of our discerning readers.

If you have any problem and also wish to seek a suitable solution to your Vaastru Shastra related problem in respect of house construction, you are most welcome to contact me direct at the undernoted address by sending a fully stamped self addressed reply paid envelop.

Office :
Agyata Darshan Complex 302
Shop No. S-1, 130 First 'A' Road,
Marudeep Apartments, Sardarpura,
Jodhpur-342003 (Rajasthan)
Phone-(Office)- 0291-637359
-(Resi)- 0291-431883
Telefax-0291-431883

PART-1
Feng Shui & Chinese Vaastu Shastra

1
What is Feng Shui?

What is Feng Shui? has become the puzzle for the common man. Indian Vaastu Shastra is based on theory of five elements and ten directions, and scholars all over the world, have acknowledged its authenticity, whereas Feng Shui is a spiritual life-style of the Chinese philosophers and thinkers and is based on the theory of Taoist religion.

Chinese convictions and beliefs are based on their own traditional thinking which has regional applicability. For instance, hanging a triple-legged frog outside a house is considered auspicious. So, one can easily find photos and idols of three-legged frog and Dragon on the shops of Feng Shui Experts. This practice is similar to Indian practice of keeping Rudraksha, Conch an Basil (Tulsi) strings of beads in the shops which sell objects relating to worship, rituals and sermons. In China Dragon is considered an auspicious animal while, we Indians call it a demon, and demons can never be auspicious. No person who indulges in meat eating and drinking is regarded as a deity.

Feng Shui and Indian Vaastu science require sustained and wide studies. Religion is the common base for both the sciences, and both firmly believe in the energies come from nature. Both the sciences also indisputably concur that such natural energies can be harnessed, utilized and made beneficial to human life.

The word 'Feng' stands for 'Wind elements' and 'Shui' for 'Water element'. Hence Feng Shui means a conglomeration of wind and water elements, but it should not be construed that Feng Shui is merely a science of wind and water elements. But the fact remains that Feng Shui also believes in the five elements, relied upon by Indian Vaastu Shastra also, but, in the context of Feng Shui, it has been used in distorted from, and we will discuss this in the subsequent chapters.

According to Feng Shui, if both the wind and water elements are combined, 'CHI' (Nature's Power) can be made more favourable. Here we have to understand the technical terminology of the Chinese language where 'CHI' is the very soul, this solitary word expressed and resembles Chinese conviction and philosophy.

Hence, in order to understand Feng Shui, we have to fully understand and digest the importance of the word 'CHI'. It is a firm belief of the Chinese that wind and water are the powerful attributes of Nature's environmental aspect, because both the elements help to sustain human life. The Chinese people believe that a person can change his fourtune, if he fully understands and strikes proper balance between these elements.

Chinese scholars align these nature's gifts with a person's daily life, chores and fortune and also align with two forms of electric energy, that is 'YIN' and 'YANG' and both the energies manage the functions of entire universe. Like an electric wire, one of these energies is positive while the other is negative can be generated, maintained and distributed when both the channels working in unison and under proper balance. Positive flow in equal quantum, from these energy sourçes paves the way to generate 'CHI'. As oxygen is the life sustaining force, similarly 'CHI' energy is indispensible for a fortunate, prosperous, life, and the energy should also flow in every dwelling unit, shop, factory and office. So, in order to fully understand the production of positive 'CHI' we have to understand the channels of energy flow properly and thoroughly. (That is, 'Yin' and 'Yang'). This aspect will be discussed in the forthcoming chapters.

In order to find convincing answers to Feng Shui posers, we have to understand the technical words which repeatedly appear and are frequently used in the Chinese language, apart from acquainting ourselves with sequence and inter relation among such words.

In order to facilitate understanding and meaning of such technical words, a glossary of such words and explanations have been appended at the end of the book so that our readers' problems, in this regard, are solved and they can easily comprehend meanings of related terms.

2
History of Feng Shui

History of Feng Shui dates back to 3000 B.C. Its origin is attributed to ancient Chinese who wanted some guidelines in respect of their land. Fields, greenery and environment. The Chinese utilised Feng Shui primarily to bury the dead bodies of their ancestors, because they firmly believe that their ancestors cast various impacts on their life. They also have a faith that a person's life and fortune can only prosper if the graves of their ancestors are placed at an appropriate site. Ancestors' soul will remain restless if their dead bodies are buried in dark graves where there are holes or in open places. They believe due to these the lives of the surviving relatives of the dead get disease-ridden and ill fortune befalls.

In Chinese civilization 'CHIN-MING' festival is celebrated once in a year. On this occasion, the Chinese offer food at the altars of their deceased ancestors and all the family members take food at the site. Such a graveyard is generally found on the southern side of the mountains so that the dead ancestors are protected from the harmful winds from the northern direction. Such graveyard on the mountains do not have any stony rocks, nor they are on uneven surface and such sites remain fully protected from burking animals and plunderers. Positive energy 'Chi' flows here uninterruptedly.

These graveyards are made in such a way that the deceased can shower blessing to their surviving relatives in their homes. These house are generally south facing, that is an entrant's face remains towards the north. There are green fields all around, and there is also provision for light, sunrays and shadow. Such houses are built in consultation with the Feng Shui master so that the house gets positive energy, 'Chi', in plenty.

The Dragon

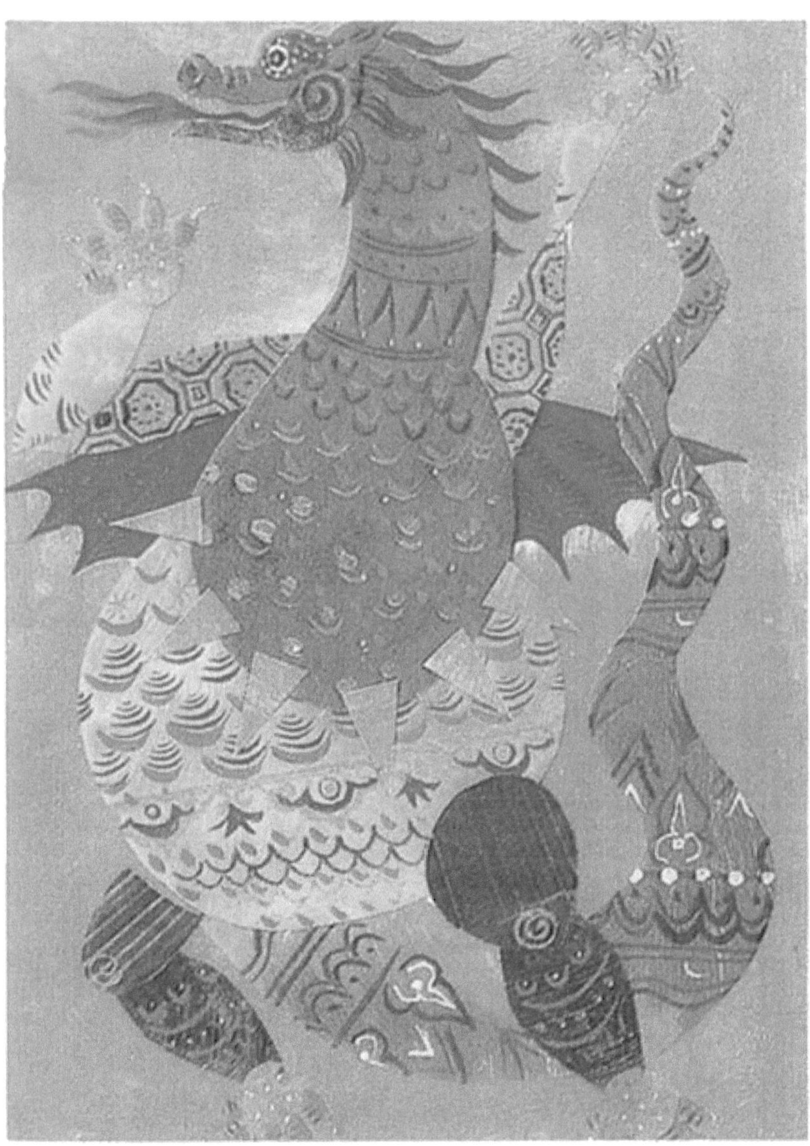

This animal belong to the species of the snakes. It can float and fly in the air, swim in the water and run at an extremely fast speed on the ground. It's paws resemble like those of the phoenix, it's body is louf like that of a snake and it emits fire from it's mouth. This animal is a symbol of strength. It's picture, at which over place dangled, will prove auspicious, as it forebodes prosperity. Hence, it is a symbol of auspicious and prosperity. It is lord of the Eastern direction.

The Black Turtle

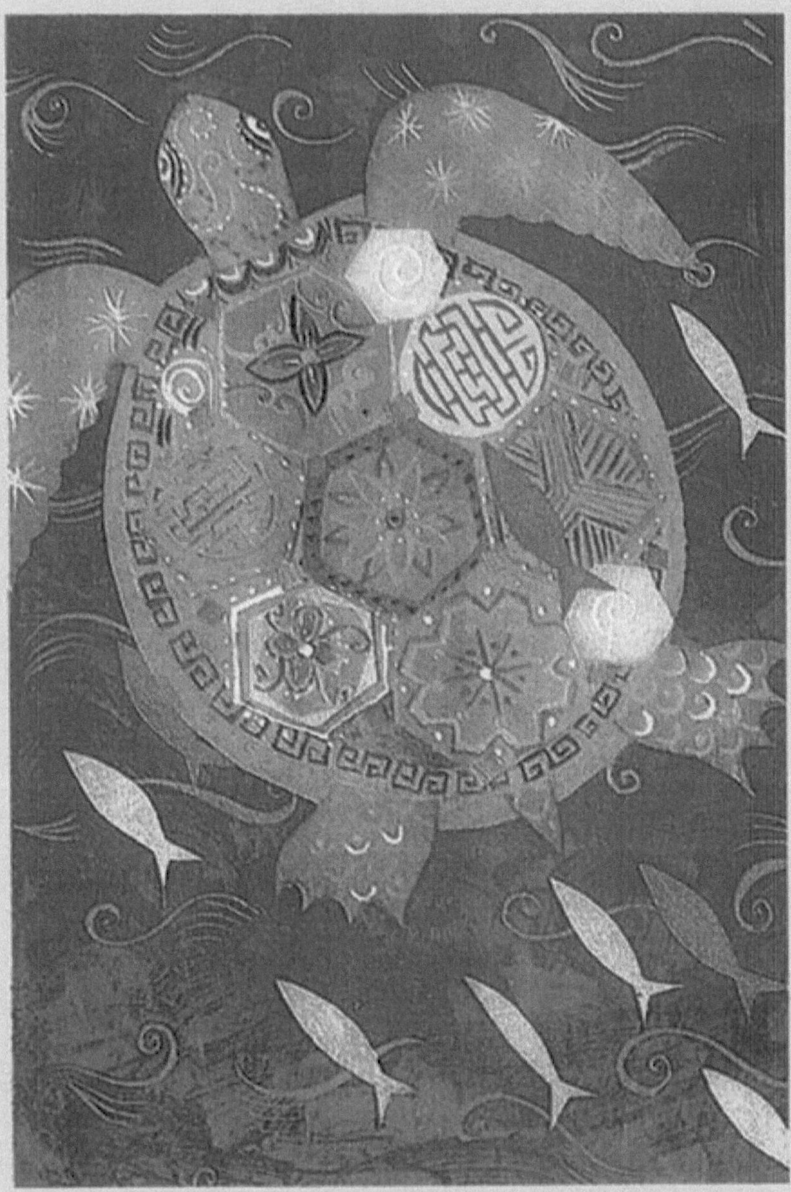

Black tortoise is considered to be the lord of the Northern direction. It is an emblem of assistance and stability. If a picture or idol of tortoise (black) is affixed towards the Northern direction, it helps to remove faults, pertaining to the Northern direction.

White Tiger

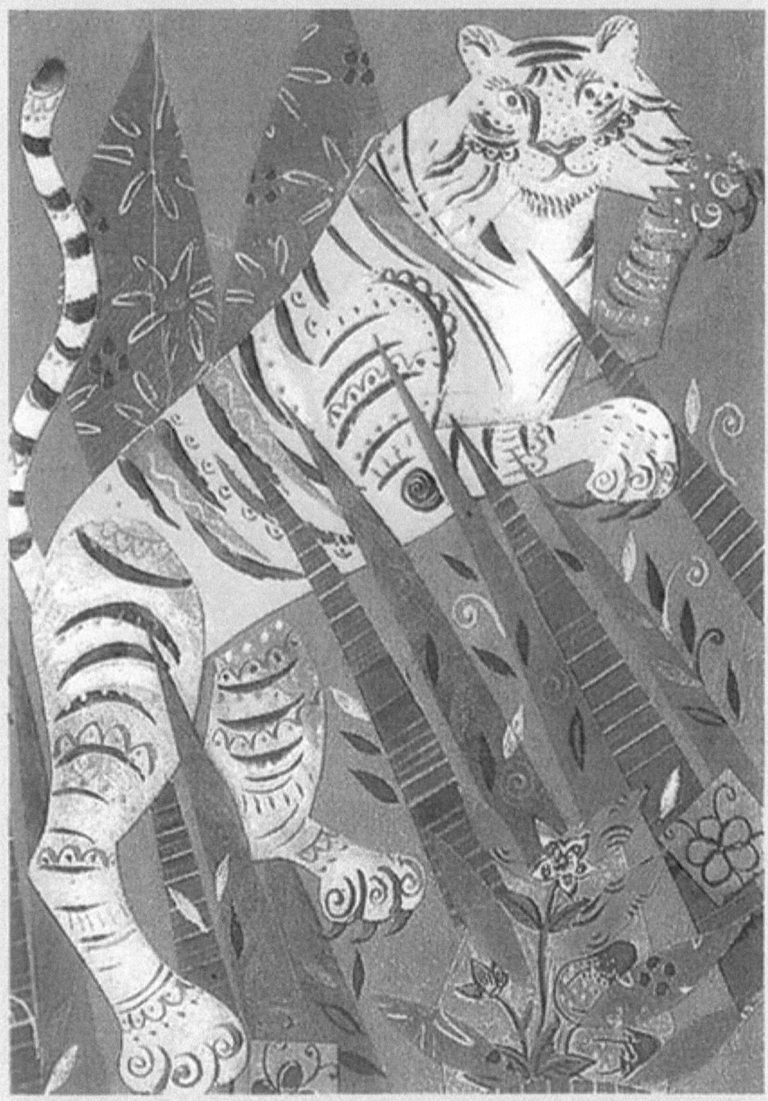

White Tiger is one of the four divine animals in Chinese astrological Feng Shui. This animal is the reigning lord of the Western direction. In order to dispel the defects, that emanate from and are related to the Western direction, it's picture is fixed on the right side of a building. It protects the house-owner from damaging impact of black magic and evil spirits.

Feng Huang

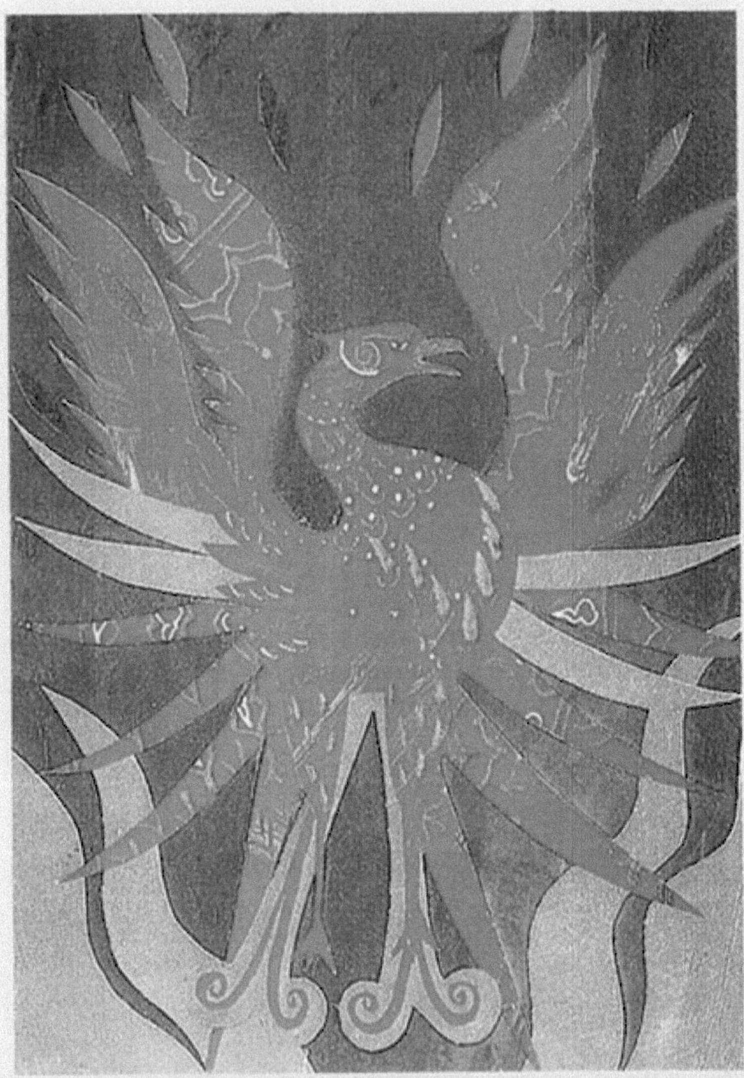

Feng Huang is a mythological bird and it's colour is red. It is the lord of the Southern direction. According to Chinese belief, pictures of this bird should be fixed on the Southern direction of the door. This is a divine bird. If picture of this divine bird or it's idol is dangled on the Southern direction of the house, it will remove Southern direction related faults and short comings and will also provide excellent opportunities to the house-owner to make progress in his life.

In addition to the above, there is also proper arrangement for discharge of stagnated and stinking water, protection from strong winds, uneven rocks, pits, disposal of urine and excreta, as all these let in harmful elements, So arrangements are made in such a way that the house remains protected from evil spirits.

A teacher adept in Feng Shui is called 'HSIEN-SHENG' and the Chinese used this word with great respect and faith. Whenever 'Hsien-Sheng' is invited to a household, a decorated palanquin is sent to bring the expert as per laid down tradition, and he is honoured and feted with great reverence. The Feng Shui expert's word is the ultimate for the household. A Feng Shui expert is a store house of natural knowledge, he wears traditional dress and decorates himself with different varieties of ribbons and laces and also supports emulates and yantras. He can suggest the type and shape of plot, method of construction in such a meticulous way that natural forces/powers help the house owner towards progress and prosperity. The Feng Shui expert guides not only about interior and exterior construction but also takes into account the atmosphere and the environs of the house.

Life on earth and wind

Signs, emblems, forms, indicators and emulets exist in abundance in Feng Shui expert analyses environs all around and suggests suitable measures. He can also sight mountain, rivers, valleys, trees and forms of various animals and analyse the inner meaning of all such aspects. Dragon is the most famous of all the animals because it is related not only to heaven, sky, water and ocean, but also to the emperors. In Chinese culture Dragon represents God's benevolence and divine power, prosperity and human's reproductive power. Dragon can appear or disappear at any place, and can assume any form, can also be seen in the form of dense clouds in the sky, as a snake in the "depths of the ocean", in the form of an insect sitting on a flower. According to the ancient Chinese belief, four large size dragons are the emperors of four corners of land beyond shores of ocean one occupying each direction.

All the crooked, high and low existing forms on the earth are the fascimiles of Dragon. The vein, within which book flows, is actually the positive energy 'Chi'. All the beautiful waterfalls, all the water evaluating resources from earth, and deep wells underneath the earth are the water-veins of the Dragon-positive energy also flows within all these objects.

In Chinese astrology, there are twelve zodiac signs and each one of these is represented by an animal, and each sign and form is indicative of various tracts of each individual sign. The Chinese have accorded these signs higher status, as each sign denotes positive import (with reference to mountains, lakes, water-falls, rivers etc). For instance, if top of any hill is conical and sharp like a pen's tip, the residents living around such a vicinity will be scholars and learned men. If people are residing in the vicinity of places, where paddy is grown, all the persons will be prosperous and

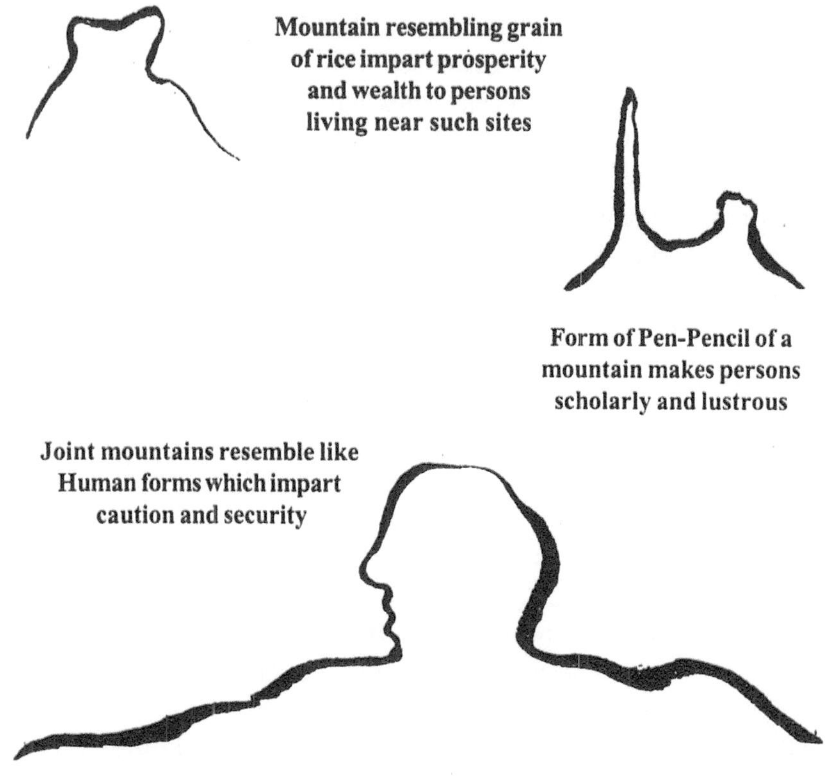

happy, because shape of rice denotes prosperity. If mountains are found in the shape of a human being, the site is indicative of some unknown power that keeps a vigil for the safety of the inmates living in such areas.

Similarly, water resources have also been accorded with great importance, because the water flowing from such natural water resources, discharges positive energy 'Chi'. That is why the shapes and forms of banks, culverts, water resources, fishes, crocodiles, dragon etc have been likened to natural symbols. In Feng Shui, such aspects were minutely examined including the land around such resources and then it was advised whether the land is worth living in. It was also studied whether the inmates living on such lands will face disaster or good fortune.

If the water dragon's role is adverse, it will invite cataclysmic situation, but, if it is favourable, it will bestow progress and profits upon inhabitants. Water Dragon's role is to cause rainfall at the most appropriate time, stop typhoons and damaging floods which devastate, and to stop occurrence of ominous events. Water Dragon yields the same respect which is accorded to the lord of water, 'Varuna' in Hindu mythological belief.

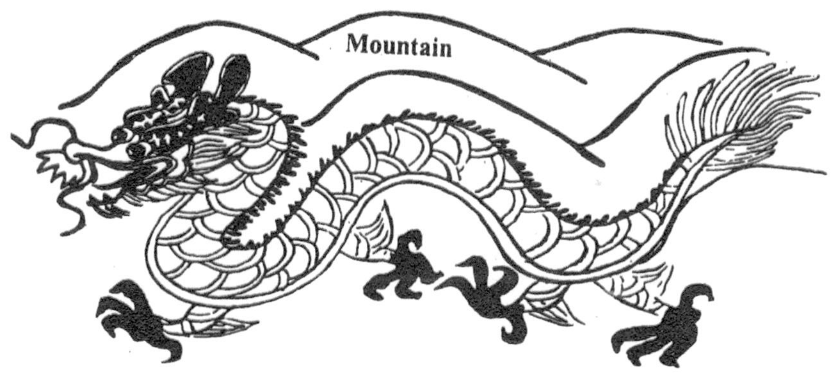

'Li' builds up congruity with life-force, and 'Chi' infuses oxygen (breath) into the same. Electric flow is activated and charged by two negative forces ('YIN' and 'YANG'). 'Chi' imparts consciousness to earth dragon by flowing through its veins and arteries. 'Chi' can abundantly be found on the summit of mountains, fast flowing water resources and water falls, and also accumulated in water ponds and slowly flowing water resources. But lakes and twined valleys restrict the flow of 'Chi', because these places are seats of 'Yin' hence, suitable for peace. Uneven and ruffled land is indicative of typhoon and darkness.

When 'Chi' flows in the rooms and other places in a house, it creates healthy and enjoyable atmosphere. Temperature and light remain fully balanced in such a house. Light 'Chi' fulfils the house with peace, prosperity, comforts and happiness.

If there is presence of 'Chi' in a house it will forestall entry of 'Sha' which is a negative energy and poses a threat to life. 'Sha' generated from filthy water-logging or foul smelling dirt. 'Sha' is also generated and generally found in natural and man-made rivers, barrages, railway lines, telephone lines, columns of trees. It casts damaging and adverse impact on the residential buildings and dwellers in such buildings suffer in their personal life.

Chinese scholars have categorised 'Chi' into the undernoted classes.

(a) Heavenly Chi

It is 'Chi' that controls and regulates cycle of seasons . During the progression and termination of four seasons, there is rise in 'Chi' and 'Yang' assumes a low profile, gradually keeps on waning, whereas during rainy season and winter 'Yin' enhances and 'Yang' goes on decreasing gradually.

(b) Growing 'Chi'

One set of spring season and light rains.

(c) Expanding 'Chi'

Pure and unhindered light, seasonal rains, onset of summer season, when grains ripe

(d) Full-grown 'Chi'

Ear-corn appear, onset of summer solstice beginning of summer season, or even completely full blown summer season.

(e) Changing 'Chi'

Onsets of winter, low heat, white drops of dew, end of winter season, 21 March or 23 September when duration of day and night is equal.

(f) Gathered 'Chi'

Snowfall, dew drops, winter season at its zenith, and light snowfall.

(g) Hidden 'Chi'

Excessive snow fall, end of winter season when duration of day and night is equal. Hidden 'Chi' is also present in slight cold and heavy rains.

3
Chinese zodiac signs and Feng Shui

As the Indians have twelve zodiac signs, the Chinese also have twelve zodiac signs (based on twelve animal signs). According to conventional Chinese treatises. Lord Buddha extended an invitation to all the animals and invited them to collect their prizes according to their individual capability. This invitation was sent on the beginning of new lunar month, but most of the animals could not make the import and purpose of such invitation, hence only twelve of the animals turned up. First of the animals to arrive was a mouse who was blessed with wisdom and intelligence. So, the first Chinese zodiac sign was allotted to mouse, then came buffalo, who was blessed with a boon of courage, and Chinese second year of zodiac circles was attributed to it. In the same pattern other ten animals came and each one of them was attributed a year each.

Though Chinese zodiac circle (rotation) differs from that of the Indian. Even then the same sign is repeated after a period of twelve years. Indian zodiac signs are based on the basis of position of such signs in the sky, where each zodiac sign can be observed, but Chinese zodiac signs are based merely on traditional legends on hearsay. Moreover, each zodiac sign in Indian astrology has its own lord (or deity) where in Chinese astrology there is no lord or any sign.

Year of birth is the most significant factor for a Chinese because any important work is done only on the basis of his birth of year. Each Chinese zodiac sign is represented by a specific animal and that animal is the symbol of a particular zodiac sign. Similary, each year, month, date and time of birth denote the qualities and traits of the concerned animal. Since each animal has specific traits, so a person born in a particular year, month and date will exhibit the traits of that animal. Also the essential five elements mould and impact the personality of the person and these are the determining factors.

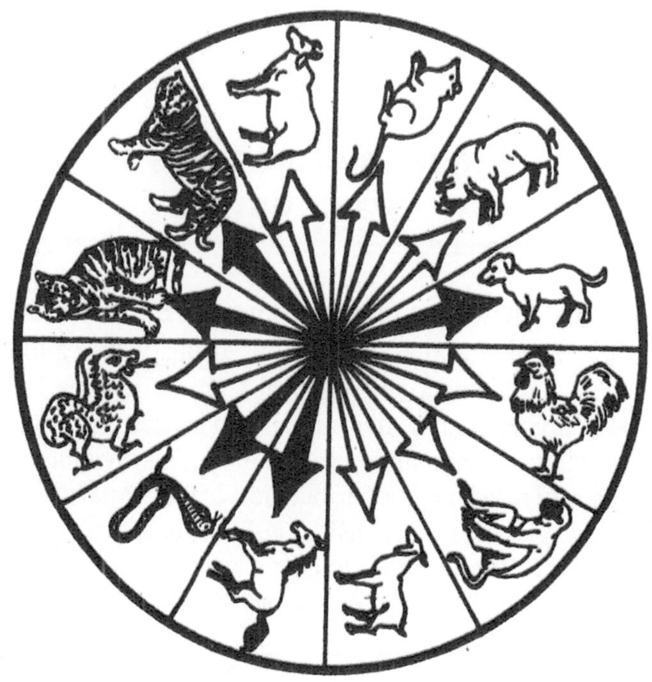

Chinese astrology is based on movement of the moon. So, the first point of significance is whether a native is born in the phase of 'God Moon' or 'Bad Moon'. All the Indian almanacs are based on Sun solstice or movement of Sun from one zodiac sign to another. The Chinese system believes in a 60-year cycle, and zodiacal belt is made up of an eighteen year celestial and heavenly stems and 12 branches of knowledge pertaining to earthly facets. Since Chinese calendar year is based on the moon, their new year starts on different dates each year. There is bound to be variation in dates in Moon and Sun based almanacs.

Sixty-year zodiacal belt has twelve earthly branches, and there are also detailed descriptions of characteristics of each of the twelve animals which invariably, denote characteristic traits of a native. Such a division of heavenly stems in ten branches is also related Yin and Yang energies. So, when Yin and Yang combine and co-ordinate with the zodiac signs and also with divine power, it is called a meeting of divine and earthly powers. Personality traits of animals are also aligned with Yin and Yang. A native's fortune and luck is formed and governed by the combination of divine and earthly powers. Years having even numbers and also ending on even numbers have Yang (positive) energy and the year ending and beginning with the odd numbers have Yin (negative) energy and their representative animals also posses positive or negative energy, in conformity and accordance with even or odd numbers-that is the reason as to why mouse, tiger, dragon, horse, monkey and jackal are positive, while cat, serpent, goat, cock, and pig are negative. Earth is Yin and heaven is Yang. So, Yin and Yang energies, even though opposite to each other, can not survive reciprocally with the aid and help of one and another. Yin is female, dark and inactive, Yang is male, bright and active. So, Yin and Yang are the energies that sustain and perpetuate existence of the world and, thus, are complementary to each other, and also stay in close proximity to each other even if their personality traits, functions and impacts are totally at variance with each other they are negative and positive wires of an electric cable. So, there is a reciprocal affinity and close relationship between the two opposite energies. Similarly, birth and death, darkness and light, day and night, heat and cold are contradictory to each other, but the existence of one can not be conceived of without the other, as each is reciprocally complementary and dependant on the other. Both are aligned to each other. Basic characteristics of Yin and Yang can be classified, as detailed here under:

YIN		YANG
1.	Female	Male
2.	Negative	Positive
3.	Soft	Hard
4.	Shadow	Light
5.	Cold	Heat
6.	Follower	Leader
7.	Wet	Dry
8.	Night	Day
9.	Earthly	Heavenly
10.	Square	Round
11.	Element	Energy
12.	In	Out
13.	Body	Soul
14.	North	South
15.	Underground	Upper Storey

The twelve Chinese zodiac signs have been segregated into four groups and each has been placed under four animals (sign). The purpose behind grouping three animals in each of the group is that persons born under the influence of these sign will have identical thinking, believe to Chinese scholars. But despite such variable facets, the style of their understanding and thinking is aligned and corresponding this common factor is the basis on which three (different) animals have been placed under one group. Let us now study the characteristic traits of animals placed in four different groups.

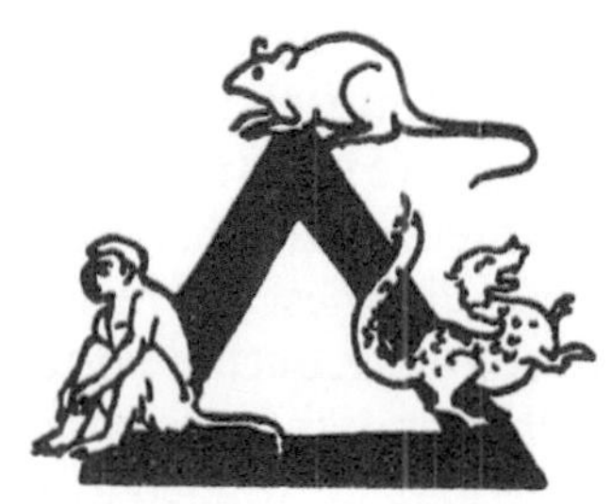

□ 1. Mouse 5. Dragon 9. Monkey

These animals, that is Mouse, Dragon and Monkey, are active animals, they have positive thinking, high class competitors and true to their character. Mouse is timid and coward, but dragon is full of courage and self-confidence, has egoistic nature and high thinking. He has the intelligence of mouse and a monkey's cunningness. It also has the ability to understand that they both can mould according to a situation. Monkey also needs intelligence of the mouse and the dragon's courage. Due to the said factors they are complementary to each other. Here mouse represents the water element, dragon the earth element and monkey the mettle element. In Indian astrology 1st, 5th and 9th zodiac signs are mutual friends because they represent the fire element.

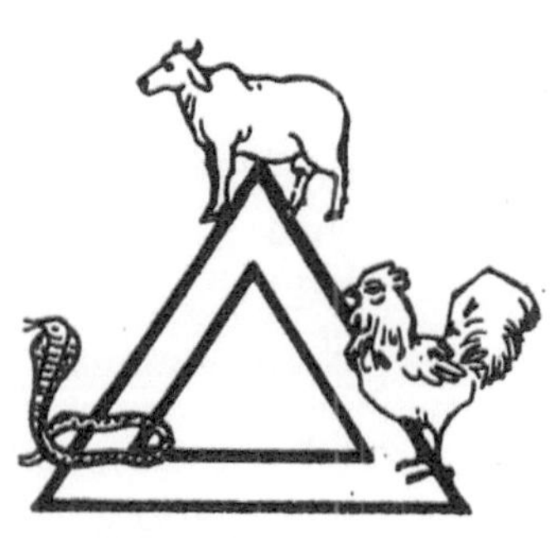

□ 2. Buffalo 6. Snake 10. Cock

Buffalo, Snake and Cock are thinkers, who always think upon one aspect or another. They are always conscious about attaining their object. Buffalo is strong and strudy, but desires to possess snake's diplomacy and attraction. The cock aspires to possess snakes alertness and buffalo's strength, and cock also wishes to posses snake's farsightedness. Here the dominant element is : Earth element buffalo, Fire element in the snake and Mettle element in the cock. But in Indian astrology 2nd, 6th and 10th zodiac signs represent each elements and are friendly zodiac signs.

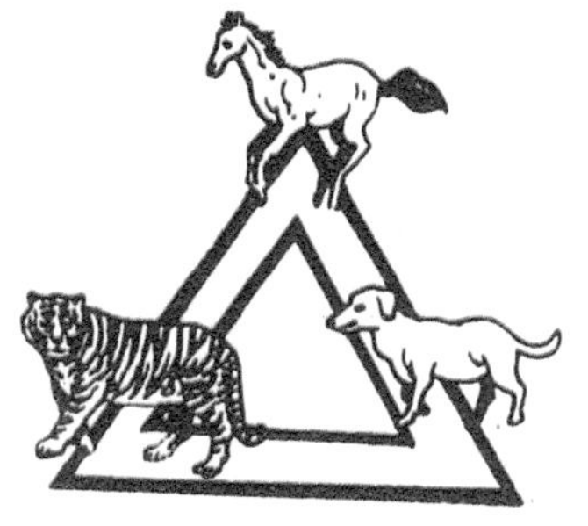

☐ 3. Tiger 7. Horse 11. Dog

Horse and Dog love freedom and hassle-free movement. These are quardrupeds and believe in situation of personal ego. Horse requires tiger's excitability and dog's transparency, Tiger needs dog's sense of duty to its master and transparency and it also need continuous mobility of the horse.

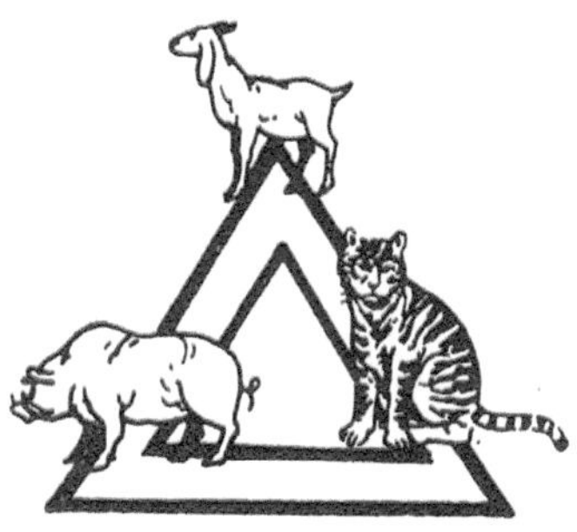

☐ 4. Cat 8. Goat 12. Pig

Cat, Goat and Pig are peace loving animals and believe in mutual co-operation. They are neither too zealous and active nor intelligent, and also do not believe in accepting challenges and risks, as they are highly sensitive creatures. They have also great ability to elicit sympathy, hence they are considerate, love and sympathise with each other. Pig requires cat's convincingness goat's civility and humility.

Here a table is given to spell out which animal is attributed to a specific month and also which is the related element.

Animal	Element	Month
Tiger	Wood	February
Cat/hare	Wood	March
Dragon	Earth	April
Snake	Fire	May
Horse	Fire	May
Goat/Sheep	Earth	July
Monkey	Mettle	August
Cock	Mettle	September
Dog	Mettle	October
Pig	Water	November
Mouse	Water	December
Buffalo (Bull)	Earth	January

Time of birth of an inmate also indicate characteristics of animals. Following table shows relation of time of birth with the related animal.

	Animal	Time of Birth
1.	Mouse	11 P.M. To 1 A.M.
2.	Bull	1 A.M. To 3 A.M.
3.	Tiger	3 A.M. To 5 A.M.
4.	Hare	5 A.M. To 7 A.M.
5.	Dragon	7 A.M. To 9 A.M.
6.	Snake	9 A.M. To 11 A.M.
7.	Horse	11 A.M. To 1 P.M.
8.	Goat	1 P.M. To 3 P.M.
9.	Monkey	3 P.M. To 5 P.M.
10.	Cock	5 P.M. To 7 P.M.
11.	Dog	7 P.M. To 9 P.M.
12.	Pig	9 P.M. To 11 P.M.

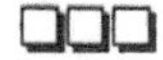

4
Chinese Zodiac Signs and Feng Shui's Elements

In order to fully understand Feng Shui, it is necessary to know exact time of birth. The sequence proceeds as follows:-

From the time of birth animal zodiac signs is determined, from the zodiac sign Feng Shui's element is determined, from Feng Shui doors of the dwelling house, bed room, study room and living room are determined.

Chinese almanac begins from the last week of January 4th or 5th February. If you are born in the month of January, you have to look for Chinese calender for the preceeding year in order to find out your zodiac sign. There are twelve zodiac signs and twelve representative symbols in both the Indian and Chinese astrological sciences but, in each system names of zodiac signs and symbols differ dramatically, which repeat in the next year in the same sequence.

For the knowledge and convenience of our discerning readers following table has been prepared which will explain Chinese zodiac signs and Feng Shui elements, from 1900 A.D. to 2020 A.D. These Feng Shui signs are taken into account while determining a native's residential and business houses, and their salient features and identification can also be ascertained.

Year of Birth	From	To	Chinese Zodiac Sign	Feng Shui Element
1900	31-1-1900	18-2-1901	Mouse	Mettle
1901	19-2-1901	17-2-1902	Bull	Mettle
1902	18-2-1902	28-1-1903	Lion	Water
1903	29-1-1903	15-1-1904	Hare	Water
1904	16-2-1904	03-2-1905	Dragon	Wood
1905	04-2-1905	24-1-1906	Snake	Wood
1906	25-1-1906	12-2-1907	Horse	Fire

1907	13-2-1907	01-2-1908	Goat	Fire
1908	02-2-1908	21-1-1909	Monkey	Earth
1909	22-1-1909	09-1-1910	Cock	Earth
1910	10-2-1910	29-1-1911	Dog	Mettle
1911	30-1-1911	17-2-1912	Pig	Mettle
1912	18-2-1912	25-2-1913	Mouse	Water
1913	06-2-1913	25-1-1914	Bull	Water
1914	26-1-1914	13-2-1915	Lion	Wood
1915	14-2-1915	02-2-1916	Hare	Wood
1916	03-2-1916	22-1-1917	Dragon	Earth
1917	23-1-1917	10-2-1918	Snake	Fire
1918	11-2-1918	31-1-1919	Horse	Fire
1919	01-2-1919	19-2-1920	Goat	Earth
1920	20-2-1920	07-2-1921	Monkey	Mettle
1921	08-2-1921	27-1-1922	Cock	Mettle
1922	28-1-1922	15-2-1923	Dog	Earth
1923	16-2-1923	04-2-1924	Pig	Water
1924	15-2-1924	24-2-1925	Mouse	Wood
1925	25-1-1925	12-2-1926	Bull	Wood
1926	13-2-1926	01-2-1927	Lion	Fire
1927	02-2-1927	22-1-1928	Hare	Fire
1928	23-1-1928	09-2-1929	Dragon	Earth
1929	10-2-1929	29-1-1930	Snake	Earth
1930	30-1-1930	16-2-1931	Horse	Mettle
1931	17-2-1931	15-2-1932	Goat	Mettle
1932	06-2-1932	25-1-1933	Monkey	Water
1933	26-1-1933	13-2-1934	Cock	Water
1934	14-2-1934	03-2-1935	Dog	Wood
1935	04-2-1935	23-1-1936	Pig	Wood
1936	24-1-1936	10-2-1937	Mouse	Fire
1937	11-2-1937	30-1-1938	Bull	Fire
1938	31-1-1938	18-2-1939	Lion	Earth
1939	19-2-1939	07-2-1940	Hare	Earth
1940	08-2-1940	26-1-1941	Dragon	Mettle
1941	27-1-1941	14-2-1942	Snake	Mettle
1942	15-2-1942	24-2-1943	Horse	Water
1943	05-2-1943	24-1-1944	Goat	Water
1944	25-1-1944	12-2-1945	Monkey	Wood
1945	25-2-1945	01-2-1946	Cock	Wood
1946	02-1-1946	21-1-1947	Dog	Fire
1947	22-1-1947	09-2-1948	Pig	Fire
1948	10-2-1948	28-1-1949	Mouse	Earth

1949	29-1-1949	16-2-1950	Bull	Earth
1950	17-2-1950	05-2-1951	Lion	Mettle
1951	06-2-1951	26-1-1952	Hare	Mettle
1952	27-1-1952	13-2-1953	Dragon	Water
1953	14-2-1953	02-2-1954	Snake	Water
1954	03-2-1954	23-1-1955	Horse	Wood
1955	24-1-1955	11-2-1956	Goat	Wood
1956	22-2-1956	30-1-1957	Monkey	Fire
1957	31-1-1957	17-2-1958	Cock	Fire
1958	18-2-1958	07-2-1959	Dog	Earth
1959	08-2-1959	27-1-1960	Pig	Earth
1960	28-1-1960	14-2-1961	Mouse	Mettle
1961	15-2-1961	04-2-1962	Bull	Mettle
1962	05-2-1962	24-1-1963	Lion	Water
1963	25-1-1963	12-2-1964	Hare	Water
1964	13-2-1964	01-1-1965	Dragon	Wood
1965	02-2-1965	20-1-1966	Snake	Wood
1966	21-1-1966	08-2-1967	Horse	Fire
1967	09-2-1967	29-1-1968	Goat	Fire
1968	30-1-1968	16-2-1969	Monkey	Earth
1969	17-2-1969	05-2-1970	Cock	Earth
1970	06-2-1970	26-1-1971	Dog	Mettle
1971	27-1-1971	15-2-1972	Pig	Mettle
1972	16-2-1972	22-2-1973	Mouse	Water
1973	23-2-1973	22-1-1974	Bull	Water
1975	11-2-1975	30-1-1976	Hare	Wood
1976	31-1-1976	17-2-1977	Dragon	Fire
1977	18-2-1977	06-2-1978	Snake	Fire
1978	07-2-1978	27-1-1979	Horse	Earth
1979	28-1-1979	15-2-1980	Goat	Earth
1980	16-2-1980	04-2-1981	Monkey	Mettle
1981	05-2-1981	24-1-1982	Cock	Mettle
1982	25-1-1982	15-2-1983	Dog	Water
1983	13-2-1983	01-2-1984	Pig	Water
1984	02-2-1984	19-2-1985	Mouse	Wood
1985	20-2-1985	08-2-1986	Bull	Wood
1986	09-2-1986	28-1-1987	Lion	Fire
1987	29-1-1987	16-2-1988	Hare	Fire
1988	17-2-1988	05-2-1989	Dragon	Earth
1989	06-2-1989	26-1-1990	Snake	Earth
1990	27-1-1990	14-2-1991	Horse	Metal
1991	15-2-1991	03-2-1992	Goat	Metal
1992	04-2-1992	22-1-1993	Monkey	Water

1993	23-1-1993	09-2-1994	Cock	Water
1994	10-2-1994	30-1-1995	Dog	Wood
1995	31-1-1995	18-2-1996	Pig	Wood
1996	19-2-1996	07-2-1997	Mouse	Fire
1997	08-2-1997	27-2-1998	Bull	Fire
1998	28-2-1998	15-2-1999	Lion	Earth
1999	16-2-1999	04-2-2000	Hare	Earth
2000	05-2-2000	23-1-2001	Dragon	Metal
2001	24-1-2001	11-2-2002	Snake	Metal
2002	12-2-2002	31-1-2003	Hare	Water
2003	01-2-2003	21-1-2004	Goat	Water
2004	22-1-2004	08-2-2005	Monkey	Wood
2005	09-2-2005	28-1-2006	Cook	Wood
2006	29-1-2006	17-2-2007	Dog	Fire
2007	18-2-2007	06-2-2008	Pig	Fire
2008	07-2-2008	25-1-2009	Mouse	Water
2009	25-1-2009	13-2-2010	Bull	Earth
2010	14-2-2010	02-2-2011	Lion	Wood
2011	03-2-2011	22-1-2012	Hare	Wood
2012	23-1-2012	09-2-2013	Dragon	Earth
2013	10-2-2013	30-1-2014	Snake	Fire
2014	31-1-2014	18-2-2015	Horse	Fire
2015	19-2-2015	07-2-2016	Goat	Earth
2016	08-2-2016	27-1-2017	Monkey	Metal
2017	28-1-2017	15-2-2018	Cock	Metal
2018	16-2-2018	04-2-2019	Dog	Earth
2019	05-2-2019	24-1-2020	Pig	Water
2020	25-1-2020	12-2-2021	Mouse	Water

Following denote related sex and direction:

Year of Birth	Male Inmate	Female Inmate
1900	North	North-East
1901	South	North-West
1902	West	North-East
1903	South-West	North
1904	North-West	South
1905	South-West	North
1906	South East	South-West

1907	East	East
1908	South-West	South-East
1909	North	North-East
1910	South	North-West
1911	North-East	West
1912	West	North-East
1913	North-West	South
1914	South-West	North
1915	South-East	South-West
1916	East	East
1917	South-West	South-East
1918	North	North-East
1919	South	North-West
1920	North-East	West
1921	West	North-East
1922	North-West	South
1923	South-West	North
1924	South-East	South-West
1925	East	East
1926	South-West	South-East
1927	North	North-East
1928	South	North-West
1929	North-East	West
1930	West	North-East
1931	North-West	West
1932	South-West	North
1933	South-East	South-West
1934	East	East
1935	South-West	South-East
1936	North	North-East
1937	South	North-West
1938	North-East	West
1939	West	North-East
1940	North-West	South
1941	South-West	North
1942	South-East	South-West
1943	East	East
1944	South-West	North-East
1945	North	North-East
1946	South	North-West
1947	North-East	West
1948	West	North-East

1949	South-West	South
1950	South-West	North
1951	South-East	South-West
1952	East	East
1953	South-West	South-East
1954	North	North-East
1955	South	North-West
1956	South-East	West
1957	West	North-East
1958	North-West	South
1959	South-West	North
1960	South-East	South-West
1961	East	East
1962	South-West	South-East
1963	North	North-East
1964	South	North-West
1965	North-East	West
1966	West	North-West
1967	North-West	South
1968	South-West	North
1969	South-East	South-West
1970	East	East
1971	South-West	South-East
1972	North	North-East
1973	South	North-West
1974	North-East	West
1975	West	North-East
1976	North-West	South
1977	South-West	North
1978	South-East	South-West
1979	East	East
1980	South-West	South-East
1981	North	North-East
1982	South	North-West
1983	North-East	West
1984	West	North-East
1985	North-West	South
1986	South-West	North
1987	South-East	South-East
1988	East	East
1989	South-West	South-East
1990	North	North-East
1991	South	North-West

1992	North-East	West
1993	West	North-East
1994	North-West	South
1995	South-West	North
1996	South-East	South-West
1997	East	East
1998	South-West	South-East
1999	North	North-East
2000	South	North-West
2001	North-East	West
2002	West	North-East
2003	North-West	South
2004	South-West	North
2005	South-East	South-West
2006	East	East
2007	South-West	South-East
2008	North	North-East
2009	South	North-West
2010	North-East	West
2011	West	North-East
2012	North-West	South
2013	South-West	North
2014	South-East	South-West
2015	East	East
2016	South-West	South-East
2017	North	North-East
2018	South	North-West
2019	North-East	West
2020	West	South-East

Hindi and Sanskrit equivalents:

South-East .... Aagneya
South-West .... Nairitya
North-East .... Ishaan
North-West .... Vaayavya

5
Detailed Description of Chinese Zodiac Signs

1. THE RAT

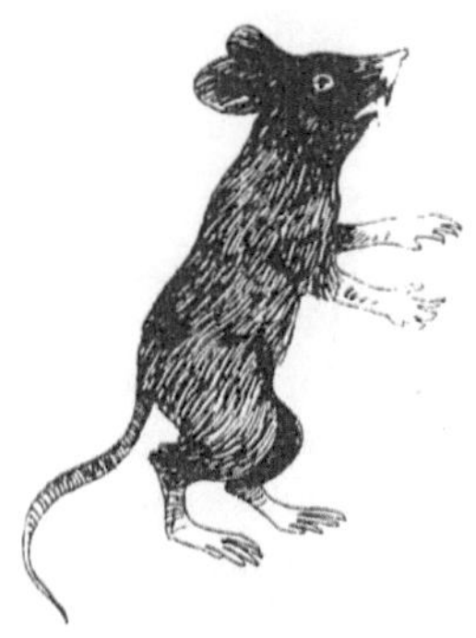

Natural Characteristic:– Intelligent and logical

Chinese Lunar Year
31 January 1900 to 19 February 1901
18 February 1912 to 06 February 1913
05 February 1924 to 25 January 1925
24 January 1936 to 11 February 1937
18 February 1948 to 29 January 1949
15 January 1972 to 03 February 1973
02 February 1984 to 19 February 1985
19 February 1996 to 07 February 1997
07 February 2008 to 25 January 2009

The Rat

This is the first zodiac sign of the Chinese. It is a predominated by water element. Those persons who are born between 11.00-1.00 p.m. (Night) have 'Rat' as their (zodiac) birth sign. Place of Rat sign stretches from 337.5-7.5 degrees in the compass and it falls under the northern direction.

Natives born under the Rat sign have attractive personality, are social and jovial. They have a sharp intellect. They pilfer food grown by other people, as they do not put in any personal labour. They take money on loan and enjoy comforts of life by using the borrowed money. They live in the realities of the present time and desire to enjoy life in the existing times. So, they do not care much for the future. They can easily make friends and feel happy in their company.

They visit clubs, parties, social gatherings and take pleasure in making arrangements for gathering and parties. Though they are laborious and also capable of envisioning good plans but, due to lack of confidence they can neither earn fame nor can they translate their plans into practical shape. They always remain restive, dissatisfied. They are competent in public relations and therefore, due to their skill in journalism and writings-this is how they come in contact with general public. Persons, whose sign is Rat, can also have lust for money, power and status. They do not spend money easily, hence they are called misers and stingy. They are quite liberal towards their friends, relatives and partners, and also are liberal towards themselves, hence they are able to pass their life with utmost comfort and convenience.

Due to lack of confidence they are timid. Their childhood passes in comfort and enjoyment, but their young age is ridden with strife and problems. Last phase of their life is quite reassured, comfortable and protected.

1. Rat and Dragon make an excellent combination

Love and marriage between men and woman of Rat and Dragon signs is by far, the most successful and excellent wedlocks. Rat is the most intelligent animal and Dragon is the strongest of the animals. Persons with Rat-sign require strength of the Dragon. Though Dragon is the most powerful animal, it lacks in intelligence when compared to the Rat. So, combination of Dragon and Rat signs is an excellent co-ordinated combination.

2. Combination of Rat and Buffalo is good

Relation and partnership between Rat and Buffalo is considered a successful combination, because buffalo is a symbol of strength, hence Rat feels perfectly secure and safe under his control and influence. When a combination of Rat and buffalo is planned, it should be ensured that freedom is not eroded or adversely impacted. Rat sign will always remain dedicated and faithful to the buffalo sign, in marriage.

3. Rat will remain dedicated towards the Monkey

Men of Rat-sign have intrinsic attraction towards the women of Monkey-sign, and the former are more inclined, dedicated and made in love for the women of Monkey-sign, whereas, Monkey women also fully enjoys with the men having buffalo-sign.

4. Horse is an arch enemy of Rat

According to Chinese' belief, horse is said to be an arch enemy of Rat, because horse's element is fire and that of Mouse is water, and enemity and hostility of fire and water elements is fully known the world over . If these signs combine, there are bound to surface squabbles and quarrels daily. Hence, it is always better of both the signs to maintain reasonable distance from each other. In other words, Men and women of Horse and Rat signs should never enter into a wedlock.

5. Snake is an enemy of Rat

A man having a Rat-sign gets attracted towards the woman having Snake-sign. There is a deep rooted natural animosity between Rat and Snake. Whenever an opportunity arises, the Snake gets provoked even at the sight of a Rat and preys on him. Hence a man of Rat-sign should always remain cautious from a woman of snake-sign, that is why both should never marry.

6. Animosity between Rat and Cat

As Snake and Rate are enemies of each other, so are Rat and Cat. They should never pull on together, because their animosity is deep rooted. Cunningness of Cat vanguishes existence of the Rat.

7. Combination of Mouse and Mouse

When both male and female have the same sign (Mouse in this context), then their dealings and nature are also identical. Both have identical aspirations. Your good behaviour and conduct will fetch you good friends, but your ill treatment and cunning behaviour will turn even your people against you.

8. Mouse and Tiger

Friendship between Mouse and Tiger is highly doubtful, because such a friendship, if at all takes place, is ridden with dangers. But if a bond of friendship can be worked out, some achievements could possibly be achieved.

9. Mouse and Goat or Sheep

Both will have ideological difference because both live an imaginary world and do not believe in physical hard work or labour.

10. Mouse and Cock

Reciprocal and mutual arguments will continue between both the signs, because Mouse is a critic and Cock-sign will also not leg behind in making futile pronouncements.

11. Mouse and Dog

Both can not pull on together, as both take interest and pleasure in disturbing each other.

12. Mouse and Pig

Both have common element in water, hence both can work out mutual friendship. Their promises to be friend, partnership in business and leading a happy married life should prove reliable. Both can also beget suddenly some new thing in life.

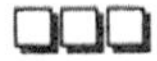

2. Buffalo

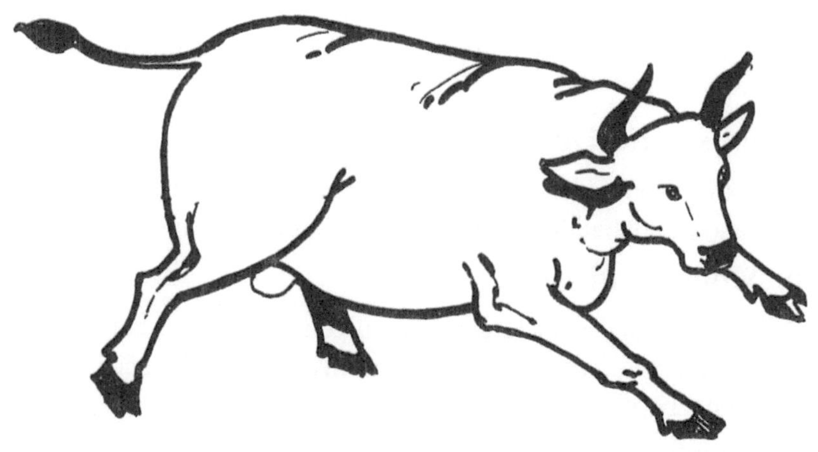

Natural Trait :– A symbol of courage

Chinese Lunar Year
19 February 1901 to 08 February 1902
06 February 1913 to 26 January 1914
25 February 1925 to 13 February 1926
11 February 1937 to 31 January 1938
29 January 1949 to 17 February 1950
15 February 1961 to 05 February 1962
03 February 1973 to 23 January 1974
20 February 1985 to 08 February 1986
08 February 1997 to 27 January 1998
26 January 2009 to 13 February 2010

The Buffalo

Buffalo is the second zodiac sign of the Chinese zodiac system and is placed in the second place, who are born between 1.00 and 3.00 a.m. have buffalo as their zodiac sign. In the compass its place stays between 7.5-37.5 degrees. Its element is earth. It represents North and North-East (Ishaan) directions. In ancient Chinese treatises, sketch of a buffalo is drawn, while in the modern books, picture or a sketch of a bull sketch ox has been drawn. In our opinion Chinese Buffalo sign has been greatly influenced by the second zodiac sign (That is 'Vrishabh' or 'Vrikha' which means an ox) of Indian zodiac system, and chance of buffalo to ox by the Chinese is simply a matter of academic interest, as both signs have identical traits and, thus different nomeclature is hardly of any consequence.

Natives of Buffalo sign are hard working, peaceful in nature but their temperament will be rash. They take pleasure in serving others. Buffalo does its works slowly, but has immense patience. At times denotes obstinacy due to which they get involved in clashes with others and difference ensue. They are labourous, self sacrificing and traditional. They have immense courage and self confidence, prefer to live in solitude. These traits are the secrets of their success. As they habitually run into age, once they get provoked, they are unable to control their anger. The buffalo (sign) is so powerful that its anger can kill even a lion with its horns, and keep on attacking the lion until he is finally dead. In 1988, I visited the thick forest of Africa and I learnt that the African people are more scared of wild buffaloes than lion, rhinoceros and elephant, because a buffalo will continue to clash and attack its (man or an animal) until it dies.

Male natives have an inborn tendency to leadership and arbitration, and none can dare stop their progress, whereas female native with a buffalo sign will prefer to live within the house than to indulge in arbitration or leadership. He wants faithfulness from all others. If he is the head of the family, his order is full and final and if his orders are flouted or disobeyed, he will consider it a crime. He can sacrifice anything to ensure that his orders are carried out entirely. He can not tolerate breach of faith and treachery.

The persons can succeed in politics and agriculture spheres, and also become successful musicians and counsellors. The Chinese believe that for a buffalo sign person, his time of birth is the most significant aspect. A buffalo native born in the winter season has a comfortable life as compared to one born in summer months. In respect of love or romance they proceed and reach the ultimate goal as they stick to their target. The Chinese also believe persons of buffalo-sign are rich.

1. Buffalo and cock were coupled in the Heaven

It is Chinese belief that buffalo-sign of male and cock-sign of female were formed in the heaven and their love emerged in the form of wedlock- it corresponds to the maxim that 'Marriages are decided in heaven, but celebrated on earth'. Both the wedded partners prefer to lead a solitary life, hence they try their utmost to make their wedded life a solitary and comfortable one. Buffalo's predominant element is earth and that of cock is mettle and it is the earth that produces mettle. So buffalo proves to be a successful partner of the women of Cock-sign, and thus their marital life is successful. Both are, thus, complementary to each other and respect the feelings of each other.

2. Snake is an intimate of Buffalo

Snakes posses attraction and the buffalo possesses strength. A native women with snake-sign has immense capacity to infatuate a buffalo male. A snake female requires a powerful and strong male, and buffalo-sign wants and needs a beautiful and attractive female. So, when both the partners join hands, it makes a happy and blissful couple. If both of them are business partners, their business will progress due to mutual understanding.

3. Variable Temperament of Buffalo and Goat

Both are temperamentally opposed to each other. Persons having buffalo-sign are sentimental, while goat-signs are not. Both have different approaches towards love affairs and life. Persons with buffalo-sign take their own decisions independently, while those of goat-sign take action after taking others in consultation. Though element of both these animals is earth, yet the Chinese scholars do not consider natives of buffalo and goat signs can make ideal and compatible couple.

4. Buffalo and Monkey

Buffalo sign gets attracted and impacted by monkey-sign. For success in life buffalo sign has to depend on monkey-sign for cleverness and power of imagination, but even then buffalo and monkey can not get along.

5. Combination of Buffalo and Tiger is dangerous

It is a famous proverb of the Chinese that persons of buffalo and tiger signs should never marry, as either of the partners is bound to die. It is also said that; if a child with lion-sign is born in a buffalo-sign person's house, the child should at once be separated from the family.

6. Buffalo and Mouse make good combination

Partnership between Buffalo and Mouse signs is said to be successful, because buffalo is a powerful animal under whose control mouse feels secure. Whenever a partnership is forged with buffalo-sign, it should be borne in mind that independence and secrecy are not intruded upon.

7. Buffalo and cat

Buffalo is strong and cat is clever, hence if both join together it will forebode a positive partnership and both will prove complementary to each other.

8. Combination of both Buffalo signs

Relation and co-ordination between two persons of buffalo-sign will prove fructuous. Both will remain in amity and co-operation unless, of course, there is some provocative an precipitatory factor.

9. Buffalo and Dragon

Both the animals have the common sign earth. Both are powerful, hence both the partners can pull on smoothly, provided there is no clash of individual ego.

10. Buffalo and Horse

Due to variable factor in approach and understanding, both the animals are liable to confrontation and collision.

11. Buffalo and Dog

There is excellent possibility of friendship between buffalo and dog. Both the animals can achieve the most when they reciprocally repose trust in each other.

12. Buffalo and Pig

Combination of Buffalo and Pig can be said to be an ideal pair. In case both zodiac signs (that is if one of the person's sign is buffalo and other's signs is Pig) both will pass their marital life with happiness and comfort.

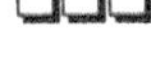

3. Tiger

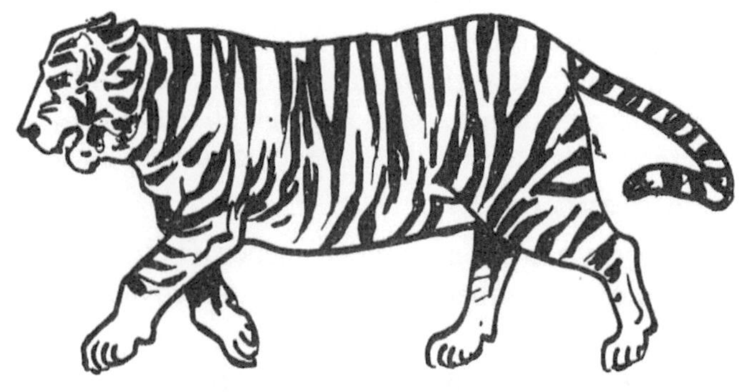

Natural Traits: Fault-finding and fiery temperament

Chinese Lunar Years						
08	February	1902	to 29	January	1903
26	January	1914	to 14	February	1915
13	February	1926	to 02	February	1927
31	January	1938	to 19	February	1939
17	February	1950	to 06	February	1951
05	February	1962	to 25	January	1963
23	January	1974	to 11	February	1975
09	February	1986	to 28	February	1987
28	February	1998	to 15	February	1999
26	February	2010	to 02	February	2011

Tiger

Tiger occupies the third place in Chinese System of Zodiac signs and its dominant element is wood. Those persons who are born between 3.00 a.m. and 5.00 a.m. have their zodiac sign, tiger. Tiger sign is situated from 37.5 to 67.5 degrees in the compass, where its place is midway to east and north-east direction.

Persons of Tiger sign are hot headed but are also courageous and active. They have high moral character, and are capable of leadership. They love to accept challenges and risks their life. They cannot be subordinates to any person. They are persons of free nature and wish to move freely. Though they are fortunate ones, but whenever they have to encounter misfortune they turn to be pessimist. They are upright and liberal persons, deceit, treachery and lying. Sometimes they fall out with their seniors and make permanent squabbles, due to their rebellious temperament, at times, situation of court cases also arises. Persons of Tiger sign are stickly, obstinate and restive, especially if they are born at night. In lovemaking they are highly sensual and beastly, but they quickly calm down also.

Generally, they have physical relations with a person of opposite sex or get married at a comparatively younger age. They will never hesitate also to stake all their belongings in love, war and gambling. The end of their life occurs suddenly under painful conditions. A native with Tiger sign is paranoide and never trust anybody. Rebellion is their natural trait.

It is a general belief in all countries that born with tiger sign persons are very fortunate and no body can match them, as they are the strongest persons on the earth. They are full of confidence. It is a famous belief of Feng Shui that where there is mortal, idol or picture of a tiger, there can not enter Thief, Fire and Evil spirits.

If there are two persons born with tiger sign, either of them has to leave the house; because tigers do not like to live in a group. First part of tiger's life is comfortable, youth period is always replete with struggle and old age is always comfortable.

1. Love between Tiger and Horse is matchless

If Tiger and Horse are bound by love their mutual understanding is unmatched. Horse's element is fire and that of tiger is wood, and it is wood that generates fire. Tiger is honest so he can easily spend his life lovingly with horse. Though they may argue for a while. Yet the arguments end on a happy note.

2. Meeting of Tiger and Dog is delightful

Marriage between Tiger sign and Dog sign indicates a happy and comfortable marriage; because both of them are fiery animals. Dog's element is earth and that of Tiger is wood, and wood grows on the earth. So both of them have identical approach to thinking and understanding, hence both get along smoothly throughout life. Similarly, partnership between tiger and dog sign can be said to be successful.

3. Beware of ladies having Tiger and Snake Signs

Persons having tiger sign should always avoid beauty and hypnosis of a lady who has snake sign, because snake being highly intelligent can not get along with the tiger. Moreover, snake's element is fire, hence her venom is also fiery.

4. Tiger and Monkey make incompatible Matching

Tiger and Monkey do not make a couple, because monkey is naughty and tiger dislikes his naughtiness. Monkey's habits are restless, and he is not trust worthy also, hence there is an hostile relation between both the signs.

5. Meeting of Tiger and Buffalo is Dangerous

It is Chinese belief and it is a maxim also that a person of Tiger element should never enter a wedlock with a buffalo element, as death of either of the married persons is a certainity. It is also held that if a child with Tiger sign is born to one with buffalo sign, the child should at once be separated from the family.

6. Tiger and Mouse

Friendship between Tiger and Mouse is always viewed with suspicion, because it is ridden with danger. But, if at all a friendship can ever be forced, it can lead to new achievements.

7. There will be continual feuds between Tiger and Cat

Though Tiger also belongs to the cat race, but cat is cleverer than the tiger and always walks ahead of him. Cat leaves back tiger on the ground and quickly scales the tree, and the tiger does not like Cat's (this) habit, because he can not live with an animal who is faster and clever than him. So, the feud between tiger and cat will continue unabated.

8. Tiger and Dragon

Friendship and partnership between tiger and dragon can last.

9. Tiger and Tiger

Even if signs of both the tiger man and woman is the same, they can not live together. It hardly matters that their breed is the same.

10. Tiger and Pig

Person having Pig sign will feel depressed and defeated in the company of person having a tiger sign, hence such thinking will prove to be a blow to their happy married life.

11. Tiger and Goat

There is an animosity between Tiger and Goat. So, a person having a goat-sign should always remain cautious, otherwise some accident can always occur at any time.

12. Tiger and Cock

Tiger and Cock signs can hardly pull on together and they should seriously look into the pros and cons before entering into a partnership.

4. Cat

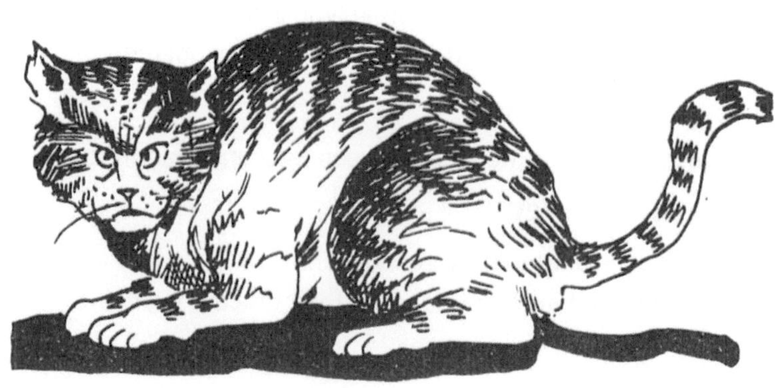

Natural Traits:– clever and cunning

Chinese Lunar Years							
29	January	1903	to	16	February	1904
14	February	1915	to	03	February	1916
02	February	1927	to	23	January	1928
19	February	1939	to	08	February	1940
06	February	1951	to	27	January	1952
25	January	1963	to	13	February	1964
11	February	1975	to	31	January	1976
27	January	1987	to	16	February	1988
16	February	1999	to	04	February	2000
03	February	2011	to	22	January	2012

Cat

Cat is the fourth zodiac sign of the Chinese system. While the ancient Chinese scholars have presented picture of the cat, modern Feng Shui experts have presented picture of the rabbit. Whoever is born between 5.00 a.m. and 7.00 a.m., gets the birth sign as cat. This zodiac sign occupies place between 67.5 and 97.5 in the Compass which is situated towards the east.

In Vietnamese literature cat sign has been substituted by the rabbit. Nature of both the animals is identical and both fall in the ground on their front paws. Cat is intelligent, clever, and worldly wise. Cat avoids quarrels and arguments. Cat succeeds in impressing people around her by sober and patient nature. Persons of cat sign are successful artists and painters, become famous in their respective fields.

Their memory is quite good. They are sociable and know fully well how to impress people whom they meet, a reason as to why they mix up freely with people at meetings, parties and gatherings. As even a wild noise alerts a cat, so the persons of cat sign always remain cautious and alert.

But their glaring weakness is they can easily be provoked by anyone against any other persons. Such natives are unreliable and can not be faithful to anyone not even to the people of their own sign, but they rely on themselves only. They can never be faithful to their master, and it would be an utmost folly to expect faithfulness from them. As for their cleverness in business is concerned, they have no competitors who can match their cleverness. Due to this quality they easily succeed in defeating their adversaries. A successful politician should preferably go in for a woman who, too, has a cat-sign, so that she also can not be defeated by anybody.

There is a belief in India and African countries that a cat and lizard takes birth in the form of a witch. Both the cat and witch drink blood. There is still a practices in vogue in some European countries that if a woman is influenced and overpowered by a cat or "wild", she is burnt alive amidst thorny bushes. The eastern countries regard cat as a sullied and unpious animal. But cat is worshipped as a goddess in Ezypt.

Cat's eyes are hotly attractive and such an attraction is also noticed in the eyes of many persons whose sign is cat. Their choicest and favourable professions are generally advocacy, shop keeping, administration or any other job where they can give vent to their sensitivity and they succeed in their work. Even though they are sociable persons, yet they remain attached to their homes. Due to their commitment to family they spend a lot of money to make the life of their home inmates more comfortable. A cat is never faithful to another of its clan. She is more conscious about her beauty. They indulge in love for the sake of only enjoyment and entertainment, but their preference is always for comfortable and hot sex relations. Natives with cat sign can reach the pinnacle of glory or attainment even by using their minimal intelligence.

1. Relationship between Cat and Goat developes gradually

Cat and goat signs are intimate friends and their friendship gradually develops and finally it strengthens into a strong bond. Earth is the element of goat and that of cat is wood. Cat sign remains faithful and committed to the goat sign. As both of them have common understanding, so both have excellent and strong marital relationship and their mutual love also remains on stronger footing.

2. Cat and Pig are made for each other

Friendship of Cat and Pig is thick and intimate. Pig's dominant element is water and cat's element is wood, and wood is saturated and nurtured by water, resultantly pig sign remains committed and dedicated to cat sign. Their meeting inspires them to do work with a spirit of "Team Work". Their marital life or practical partnership and mutual love are so strong that both can be said to be made for each other.

3. Cat and Dog

Cat and Dog may pull on together but, for their inherent and natural animosity they can fall out, because animosity will be the cause of feud, hence utmost caution is necessary.

4. Cat and Mouse are enemies

Cat and Mouse can not pull on together due to inherent mutual animosity. Similar is the case with Cat and Rabbit. They are born adversaries and their animosity is deep rooted. Whenever the cat seizes an opportunity she puts to end the existence of the mouse.

5. Strife between Cat and Tiger is an on going process

Tiger also belongs to the cat race, but the cat is far clever is and cunning then the tiger. Cat leaves a tiger in the lurch, but herself climbs the trees, thus leaving the latter to feud for himself. This habit of the cat is not liked by the tiger, because he can not pull on or make amends with an animal who is clever and faster than him. So, a feud between the cat and tiger will continue infinitely.

6. Cat and Snake

Their inherent animosity reaches its zenith, because cat's element is wood and that of snake is fire and it is the fire that turns wood into ashes, snake's venom is poisonous which is fatal for the cat. So, both the signs can not see eye with each other, hence incompatible.

7. Cat and Buffalo

Buffalo is a strong and powerful animal whereas cat is clever. So, they are complementary to each other and also that they can make successful partners married couples. They will also make their future bright.

8. Cat and Dragon

From spiritual view point, meeting of cat and dragon is incompatible.

9. Cat and Cat

A person of cat sign will hate another person whose sign is also cat.

10. Cat and Monkey

Cat and monkey sign can not pull on together.

11. Cat and Cock

These have born and inherent animosity.

12. Cat and Horse

If both have identical understanding they can pull on, otherwise not.

5. Dragon

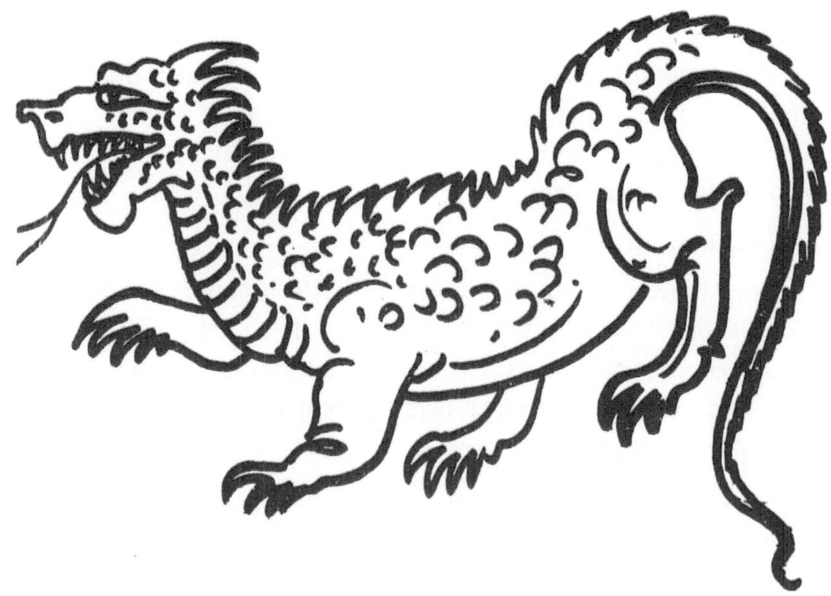

Inherent Trait:– Proud and courageous

Chinese Lunar Years						
16	February	1904	to	04	February	1905
03	February	1916	to	23	January	1917
23	January	1928	to	10	February	1929
08	February	1940	to	27	January	1941
27	January	1952	to	14	February	1953
13	February	1964	to	02	February	1965
31	January	1976	to	18	February	1977
17	February	1988	to	05	February	1989
05	February	2000	to	23	January	2001

Dragon

Dragon is the fifth zodiac sign in Chinese astrological system. Its elements is wood. Persons born between 7.00 am and 9.00 am. have their birth signs as 'Dragon'. This sign lies between 97.5 and 127.5 degrees on the Compass. Its area falls between east and south-east direction.

Dragon is a symbol of good fortune. The Chinese consider the Dragon year as the best and most fortunate, because the persons born under this sign are extremely intelligent, fortunate, healthy, lively, imaginative and strong-willed. Due to these qualities they achieve their goals which they set out for themselves, People having a dragon-sign have an extrovert personality and possess a strong will power. They can easily attract others due to their show off. They can easily face all the odd situations quite easily. They always wish to remain popular, but they can not be easily influenced by others nor they can be taken in easily.

If they turn animical and hostile, their animosity assumes seriousness and dangerous proportions, though generally they are quite gentle and helpful friends. Any fact of life where they can get publicity are the best suited situations for them. So, they are highly successful in politics, military, religious organisations where they can get publicity. Persons having a dragon sign at a much later stage, that is when suitable time for the marriage has already run out. Some time they remain unmarried also. Due to their habit of living in solitude. There is an element of dissatisfaction in love. They resort to polygamy or indulge in adultery.

Persons born in dragon sign believe in outward pomp and show. They are naughty reason as to why dragon woman remain always surrounded by their admirers.

Dragon people emerge successful wherever they go or take up any work. They are talkative and out-spoken and weave a delusive and illusive atmosphere around them and create an unrealistic environment.

Dragon is considered a symbol of extreme spiritual power in China and entire Asia. They believe that if one keeps its picture or idol it will bring in four things (virtues), that is, wealth, good habits and virtues, ostentation and comforts and long life since dragon has an inherent power and ability, the people having dragon sign, can easily guess what idea lies in another person's mind.

In China, dragon is considered as a pious animal, but in India and eastern countries, it is considered a demon; hence they reject this animal. It resembles a dangerous lizard or a flying viper, hence its description matches with the description of demons mentioned in the Puranas. But in Feng Shui a Dragon is regarded as an emblem of natural positive power (energy), and that's why the Chinese consider it adorable, powerful animal fit to worship.

1. Dragon and Mouse combine ensures spiritual happiness

According to Chinese beliefs, marriage between dragon and mouse signs is indicative of a spiritual union. As dragon is blessed with power and mouse with intellect, hence reciprocal meeting of both the signs ensures comforts and prosperity, because both complement each other. Element of mouse is water and that of dragon is earth, and it is the water that imparts reproductive capacity to the earth. Dragon is an animal having a large body and Mouse is an animal of a tiny frame, so mouse always feels softened secure under dragon, Mouse can also submerge from under the dragon's imposing personality. Due to the said factors combination mouse and dragon signs is considered the most appropriate couple.

2. Dragon and Monkey's love is ideal

Dragon and Monkey are considered to be intimate friends. When monkey's ambition and dragon's power join together, there is an emergence of superior and excellent love. Monkey's element is mettle and dragon's element is earth, and mettle is a productive of earth. When monkey and dragon signs meet they can succeed in giving birth to alternative children.

3. Attraction between Dragon and Snake

A dragon man always gets attracted by a snake woman. His joy knows no bounds when a dragon gets married to a beautiful snake woman who keeps dragons vanity under control by her entertaining and relaxed nature. Their conduct helps each partner to maintain and enhance attraction mutually towards each other.

4. Dragon and Cock

Love marriage between dragon and cock signs is quite possible and their marriage is also successful, because they can manage to pull on together of course with mutual cooperation and understanding. Women having cock sign generally puts on weight after their marriage.

5. Dragon and Tiger

Relationship between dragon and tiger will always remain feud ridden because both of them are extremely haughty and arrogant.

6. Dragon and Buffalo

Dragon and buffalo have earth as their elements. Both are powerful also. Hence if there is no clash of ego, their married pair will be in order and can also pull on well.

7. Dragon and Dog

Dragon and dog are arch enemies. The Chinese firmly believe that either a marriage or a partnership between dragon and dog signs will not be compatible.

8. Dragon and Pig

There is a possibility of meeting between the Dragon and the pig signs as both can pull on together, but in doing so the pig sign has to sacrifice more, dragon is more dominant and powerful of the two.

9. Dragon and Goat

Since general conduct of both the dragon and the goat is identical, they can forge an alliance but there will be neither gain nor loss. It is imperative that the relevant factors are carefully matched and then decided.

10. Dragon and Dragon

Both the dragon man and dragon woman can be tied in a wedlock and their marriage will also be auspicious and comfortable, as both the partners firmly believe in outward show off.

11. Dragon and Cat

From the spiritual view-point meeting of dragon and cat is incompatible.

12. Dragon and Horse

Element of dragon is dominated by earth, while that of horse is fire. But, even then, there is some similarity between the two signs. Both are emblems of strength, both are attractive and fast. Hence dragon and horse can pull on perfectly well. If the horse-sign remains committed and dedicated to the dragon sign, partnership between both the signs can be productive and successful.

6. Snake

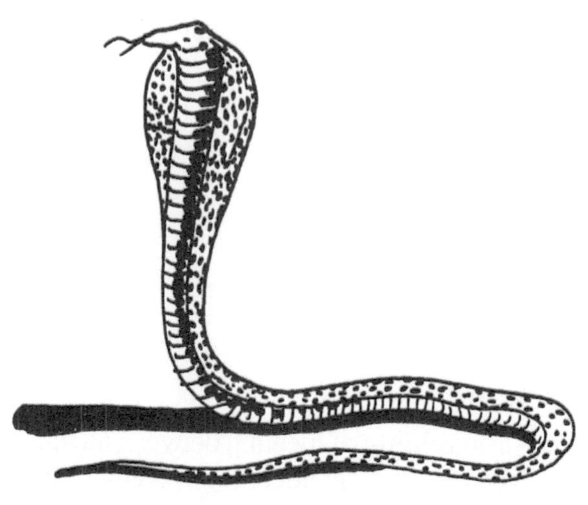

Natural Trait:– Hypnotist and a natural charmer

Chinese Lunar Years						
04	February	1905	to	25	January	1906
23	January	1917	to	11	February	1918
10	February	1929	to	30	January	1930
27	January	1941	to	15	February	1942
14	February	1953	to	03	February	1954
21	February	1965	to	21	January	1966
18	February	1977	to	07	February	1978
06	February	1989	to	26	Jnauary	1990
24	January	2001	to	11	February	2002

Snake

Snake occupies the sixth place in Chinese zodiac sign and its element is fire. Persons born between 9.00 a.m. and 11.00 a.m. will get Snake as their sign. This sign occupies 127.5 to 157.5 degrees in the compass. Its direction is east and south-east.

The western world, especially the Christian community, regards snake as a devil. But Snake is worshipped as a deity in India where it is known as 'Naag Devata'. In China, a person born in the snake sign is considered wealthy. Women, with the snake sign are extremely beautiful. They are blessed with intelligence, calmness, sobrity and wisdom. Their brain always remains active in plans. Persons with snake sign are serious thinkers, capable to accept challenges, but they have an unsteady mind. This is the reason why they take longer to decide on important matters. Their temperament is authoritative, hence when their feelings are ignored, they turn jealous. Men and women, whose sign is snake, put on very attractive clothes. They are persons of jovial and entertaining nature, they never waste away their time in useless pursuits, nor do they indulge in loose talk. They are intrinsically introverts. Their habit to live in loneliness sometimes creates hurdles in their way of establishing contact. Their confidence, will power and capacity to think help them to attain success, hence they gain popularity quite easily.

If, however, they fail in achieving their objectives in life, they take long to overcome the disappointments. If they are challenging, they retaliate by taking revenge. Persons of snake-sign can suffer from high blood pressure and nervous diseases. They can ably discharge duties as teachers, managers and social advisors. They faithfully and successfully discharge the work assigned to them. They are extremely choosy and selective in love and will never compromise on their perferred choice. They are also very jealous. In case of money they are fortunate, but they do not spend lavishly. They help others not by giving money but by helping them in person.

Snake is also called a miniature dragon, people of snake-sign can take quick decisions. In order to achieve their goal they will burn midnight oil and keep no stone unturned. They will take respite only after they have achieved their goal.

These persons have a large family because they believe in producing more children. Persons of snake-sign are luckier if born at mid-day of summer, whereas those born at night in winter are not that lucky. But if a native of snake-sign is born during a typhoon-ridden night he proves very harmful for the society and his personal life becomes also full of challenges.

1. Snake and Cock are intimate friends

According to Chinese belief, there is an intimate friendship between the signs of snake and cock, and it turns their love-affair into an ideal marriage. People of the cock sign are appreciative of the style of working and way of thinking of people of the snake sign. Snake gives a suitable advice and cock acts upon such an advice. They are excellent complementaries to each other due to which their marital life is extremely successful, as they pull on well together. Cock's element mettle and that of the snake is fire. Fire melts metal, due to this factor, cock will always remain dedicated and committed to snake's love.

2. Snake and Buffalo are best friends

Snake is attractive and buffalo is powerful. A snake woman intensely attracts and fascinates a buffalo, because a snake woman requires a strong buffalo sign man and buffalo-sign man also requires a beautiful snake-sign woman. So meeting of the both is considered joyous, comfortable and complementary. If both are partners in business, their business will progress due to good mutual understanding.

3. Snake and Pig

If snake and Pig signs marry, then snake will dominate over upright and steadfast Pig. A lady with snake sign will continue to represent the man having pig-sign for his short-coming. But if the lady has a pig-sign she will patiently and delightedly continue to listen her partner having a pig sign, and manage to pull on. Their marriage can not said to be an ideal one due to their variable elements, as snake's element is fire and that of pig is water-water extinguishes fire and fire heats up water.

4. Snake and Tiger

Men having tiger-sign should be cautious and beware of girl born under the sign of snake. They should not be influenced by snake woman's beauty because they can not pull on together because of cunningness of the snake. Moreover, snakes's element is fire and its fire is venomous also.

5. Snake and Mouse

Mouse gets easily fascinated by a woman of snake sign, though they have inherent animosity which is quite deep rooted also. When an opportunity arises, the snake gets provoked and preys the mouse. Hence man of mouse sign should remain cautious from a woman whose sign is snake.

6. Snake and Cat

There is inherent animosity between snake and cat, cat's element is wood and that of snake is fire and it is well known that fire burns wood, therefore snake's venomous fire is also fatal for the cat. Hence no relationship is possible between them.

7. Snake and Dragon mutually fascinate each other

Dragon male always gets infatuated and attracted by the beauty of a snake woman, and his joy knows no bounds when he establishes relation with a snake woman. Due to her jovial entertaining temperament snake woman proves instrumental in putting down and controlling arrogance of the dragon, so their mutual conduct and behaviour instils a sense of joy between them.

8. Snake and Snake

Snake-sign believes in adding to the number of its children which is its natural and traditional trait, hence man and woman of snake-sign are mutual friends. They do not also have any intrinsic, but personal animosity or friendship will depend on their nature and temperament.

9. Snake and Horse

Element of both the snake and horse is fire and both are provocative and attractive. Hence if the snake accepts the superior power of the horse, both will revel in love and their love will extend. If the snake-sign is dedicated, it will be excellent for a marriage.

10. Snake and Goat

Both the signs will love each other, but goat-sign should always remain cautious about snake's cleverness.

11. Snake and Monkey

Meeting of snake and monkey is a meeting of fire and mettle elements. Hence there is no natural animosity between them. If both the sign have natural understanding and sympathy they can pull on happily and nicely.

12. Snake and Monkey

Both snake and monkey represent the fire element. So their friendship is also natural. If natural understanding and consideration is there, they can lead a happy life.

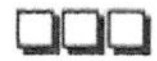

7. Horse

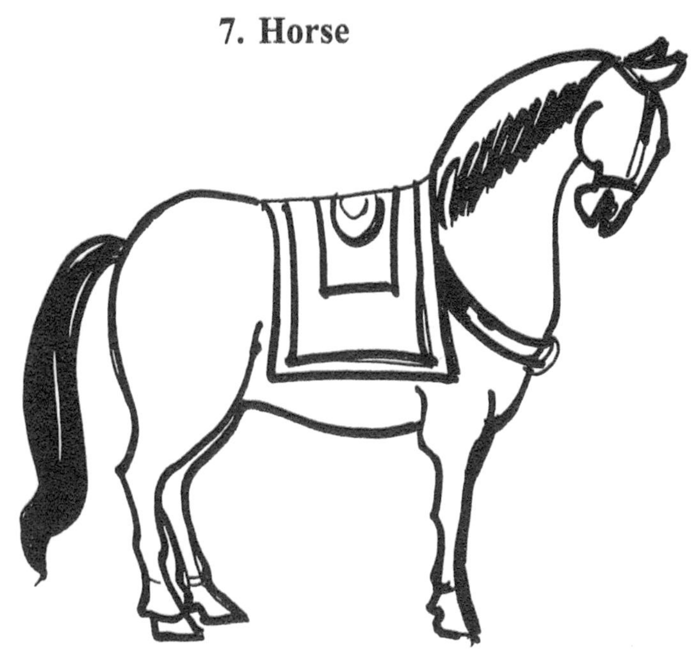

Natural Trait: Mobility, activity and attraction

Chinese Lunar Years							
25	January	1906	to	13	February	1907
11	February	1918	to	01	February	1919
30	January	1930	to	17	February	1931
15	February	1942	to	05	February	1943
03	February	1954	to	24	January	1955
21	January	1966	to	09	February	1967
07	February	1978	to	28	January	1979
27	February	1990	to	14	February	1991
12	February	2002	to	31	January	2003

Horse

Horse is the seventh zodiac sign in the Chinese zodiacal circle and its element is fire. Persons born between 11.00 a.m. to 1.00 a.m. have horse as their birth sign. The horse sign occupies 157.5 to 187.5 degree in the Chinese compass. It is placed in the southern direction.

Horse sign is sociable and the persons whose birth-sign is horse love freedom social relations. They are adept in the art of influencing people. They are always at the centre of attraction. They have in born quality of leadership and their magnetic personality plays an important role. Persons of Horse-sign are appreciated for their frankness and honesty. They take part in thoughtful deliberations and discussion, and keep themselves engaged in one activity or another. But being persons of independent nature, they do not bind themselves with rules and regulations which they actually hate. Like those born with the snake sign such persons take long time to recover from the shock of failures. They have sharp intellect, labourious and hard working. They are adept in earning money and that's the reason why they always find finance as a convenient and suitable profession. They not only earn money but also gain power and fame.

Persons born with horse as their birth-sign easily and quickly established love relations. But they love only for their selfish motives and, if they fail in their love affairs, they take such failures in normal stride and do not get depressed. Due to their sharp intellect they are able to take quick and instant decisions. The biggest stumbling block is their drawback of hot headness and impatience. They easily and quickly get enraged and will not forgive their adervsaries. They also can not be subservient to anybody nor can they tolerate being bossed by anyone. They can succeed in business only when they work independently , because subservience renders them weak.

Persons with horse-sign are short tempered. Their mood keeps on changing. If they have faith in person, they will sacrifice everything for him. They are obedient and committed to their mother and wife. Opposite sex is their weakness, so they remain dedicated to the member of the opposite sex.

Fire Horse

Normally Horse-sign re-emerges automatically after a span of twelve years, but after a period of sixty years 'Fire Horse' enters the 'Horse' Sign' which in Chinese parlance is an event of great importance. The years

1906, 1966 and 2026 are thought to be the years of Fire-Horse and these years are extremely significant due to its greater powers than the ordinary Horse. It fame spreads like the flames of fire. This famous name is allotted to a famous Chinese. But such a person's birth is considered as ominous for his family.

1. Horse and Dog relationship till final moments

Marriage between persons born with horse and dog is thought to be auspicious, and family life remains strong and long lasting, say upto the end of life. If the male has a horse as birth sign the person with dog sign to listen to and understand him. Horse is ambitious and dog gets pleased by his success. So, they reciprocally remain happy and satisfied with each other. Their partnership succeeds and pulls on well, as both are complementary to each other.

2. Horse and Tiger make excellent combination

Both horse and tiger are symbols of strength. They are hard-working. They love independence, move freely and believe in taking risks. Since their thinking alike, they will make an excellent couple. As element of the horse is fire and that of the, tiger is wood, and it is the wood that generates fire, hence tiger will remain dedicated to the horse. There is also reciprocal affinity between the elements.

3. Horse and Snake

Both the horse and snake have fire as common element, both are provocative, (stimulant) and attractive. So, if the snake reconciles to and accepts power of the horse, they will make a matchless pair. Further, if the snake-sign remains dedicated to the horse they will make a successful and loving married couple.

4. Horse and Mouse

According to the Chinese belief, horse is the first rank arch enemy of mouse. Horse's element is fire but that of the mouse it is water. And enmity between fire and water is a universally accepted. Whenever these signs come in to contact, there will be squabbles, so, it always better that both stay clear of each other, because they can never pull on together.

5. Horse and Pig

Horse's dominant element fire and that of pig is water there is mutual enmity between the two. The horse is a fast animal but pig is a simpleton. There is also variance in mental approach between the two. Moreover their speed of activity is also at variance, hence will be a blunder to match natives born with these signs as they can not live under one roof.

6. Horse and Buffalo

Thinking and approach of both the animals sign is diametrically opposite to each other, hence there is bound to be a confrontation between the two, whenever they meet.

7. Horse and Cat

If both the signs can reciprocally reconcile and understand each other, they fully come together, otherwise not.

8. Horse and Dragon

Earth is a predominant element of the dragon and that of horse is fire. There are same common attributes between the two signs-both are symbols of strength, both are fast and attractive also. Hence dragon and horse can ably put on nicely. If horse-sign remains dedicated and faithful to dragon-sign, in that even their partnership can be beneficial and fruitful.

9. Horse and Horse

There is a natural affinity and love between both persons if born with horse sign. Because both belong to the same breed, and being a social animal, horse loves to live in company of other horses. So, if a man and woman has a common sign with horse, both will pull on nicely.

10. Horse and Goat

Horse's element is fire and of a goat is earth principally they are congruent. But goat has to sacrifice, remain dedicated to horse, only then the former can pull on with the later. If it is so, then only both can continue with their family life and partnership.

11. Horse and Monkeys

Element of horse is fire and that of monkey is mettle. So both have principally the same equality, due to this factor both can pull on together.

12. Horse and Cock

Horse's element is fire and earth is the element of cock, hence both have element equality, but the horse is powerful and cock is an animal with weak will power. If the cock remains dedicated to the horse, the pair's marriage will be successful and also of that their partnership will also be productive.

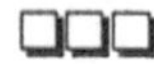

8. Goat

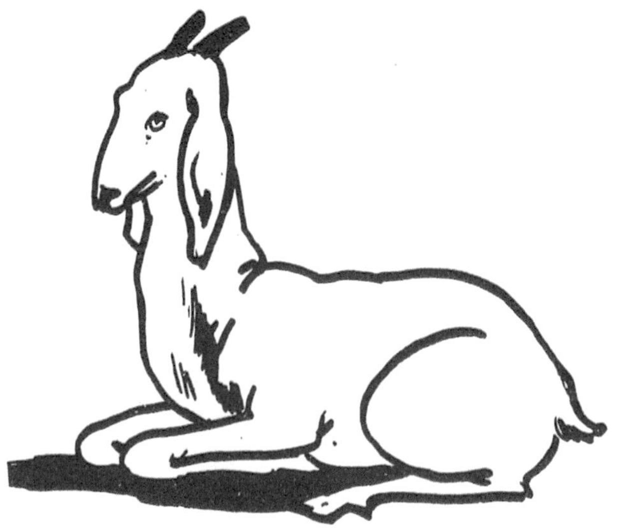

Natural Trait: Obedient and Follower

Chinese Lunar Years						
13	February	1907	to	02	February	1908
01	February	1919	to	21	February	1920
17	February	1931	to	06	February	1932
05	February	1943	to	23	January	1944
24	January	1955	to	12	February	1956
09	February	1967	to	27	January	1968
28	January	1979	to	15	February	1980
15	February	1991	to	03	February	1992
01	February	2003	to	21	February	2004

Goat

Goat occupies eighth place in Chinese Zodiac circle and its element is earth. What the ancient Chinese scholars called as 'Goat' has been changed to 'Sheep' by the modern Feng Shui experts and each one of whom has also included figure (5) of 'Goat' and 'Sheep' in their respective descriptions. The change of approach seems to have been influenced by 'Mekha Rashi' of Indian zodiac system. Persons born between 1.00 am and 3.00 p.m. have their zodiac sign as 'Goat'. It occupies a place between 187.5 and 217.5 degrees in the compass. Its place lies in between the southern & south-west ('Nairitya of Vaastu') directions.

People with Goat sign are lovers of art, perform constructive work. They can also do business in the said disciplines and can be successful. They are civilized and cultured and have great respect and consideration for feelings and comforts of others. Temperamentally they are calm and quite but love to live in solitude, hence they do not like crowds and crowded places. They prefer to lead a comfortable and hassle free life, free from tension and disturbance. They can not lead a roped daily routine nor can they start to a routine schedule, where there are too many conditions attached.

Women of Goat-sign wish to marry wealthy men. They require a strong man to motivate them and take the best out of them. When people of goat-sign are criticized, they take such criticism on personal level and also react strongly to it.

They prove to be excellent partners, as they leave the decision (to be taken) to their partners and then forge towards their avowed goal. Their instant reaction to cirticism leads them to despondency. Knowledge about art is their natural trait, hence they can prove their capability to the optimum limit in the field of art, music, plays etc.

By birth and intrinsically they are persons of constructive nature, but they require proper inspiration and direction. They have intimate relations with those persons who are less sensitive and strong in temperament. Due to their good fortune they are lucky in not facing any monetary crunch, rather paucity of feuds is never their worry. But at times they can throw discipline to winds and also be irresponsible. Their weakest point being that they can never be serious about their responsibilities, since they hate wars, they do not like any job in army and police.

Persons of Goat-sign are dual-natured. They always try to appease their enemies and friends in the same breath. They are reckoned as the leading personalities in their society. They are born to carry out orders of other persons and follow footsteps of their leaders. If other planetary positions are favourable they might become second grade leaders. They remain behind the scene but are led by someone else, that is they are not front-runners but only back-benchers.

Goat is a female sign, and men of Goat-sign bleat like the goat or sheep, but they can not roar like a lion. They have no independent thinking or philosophy. Hence, act as per the advice of other persons. They can not also labour hard nor they have the capacity and courage to face others.

1. Love between Goat and Pig is undescribable

Bond of love between Goat and Pig can not be described in words. Goat feels happy lucky and privileged to be loved by selfless love of the Pig. Goat's element is earth and that of Pig is earth, and it is the water that impacts fertility and reproductivity to the earth. Hence when goat and pig meet, they can give birth to the best quality of children. Everyone of them is happy to perform job for the other partner. Hence, marriage, love relation and partnership between both the signs is permanent and everlasting.

2. Love between Goat and Cats is like resounding of sweet musical notes.

In Chinese treatises love between goat and cat is considered to be an excellent one. Goat's element is earth and cat's elements is wood, and wood grows on earth; hence wood is a bi-product of earth. Hence cat is the assisting factor/element for the goat. Cat is a nurturer and goat is a simpleton animal. When simplicity and cleverness join hands, it forges an excellent situation for a happy, comfortable and prosperous marital life. There is also plenty of mutual understanding between both the signs.

3. Variable Temperaments of Goat and Buffalo

There is an ocean of variation between the temperaments of goat and buffalo, because people of buffalo-sign are sentimental, while those of goat sign are not. Further, people of buffalo sign take their decision on their own, while those of goat-sign follow the advice of other people, and is guided by them, though earth is a common element of both the animals, yet the Chinese scholars do not consider relations between buffalo and goat as practical and suspicious.

4. Goat and Horse

Element of the horse is fire and that of the goat is earth, and elemental recognition also exists between them, but, even then, Goat-sign has to make sacrifice and remain dedicated so that it could pull on with the horse-sign it is a prerequisite for a smooth running of marital life and partnership.

5. Goat and Dog

Even though there exists elemental similarity between both the animals, yet they can not pull on together, due to natural enmity between them. So, both can not pull on under one roof.

6. Goat and Goat

Meeting between men and woman is possible as their sign is identical. Both believe in living, grazing and digging together. Moreover, they are not generally seen quarrelling with each other unless, of course, there exists some grave danger. Though women of the goat-sign can remain together, but relation between men and women of the same sign will be feud-ridden and arguments could also follow.

7. Goat and Mouse

Both the animals will continue to have ideological differences, because both dwell in an imaginary world and also generally slum physical labour.

8. Goat and Tiger

Both are natural enemies. Persons of goat sign should always remain vigilant and guarded due to tiger's demeanour, otherwise chances of mishap might occur.

9. Goat and Dragon

Behaviour of goat and dragon is on an equal-footing-there is neither any gain nor loss, But extra caution is required while tallying both signs.

10. Goat and Snake

Though there will be reciprocal affinity between both the animals yet the goat-sign should remain cautiously guarded from the treacherous habit of the snake-sign.

11. Goat and Cock

Cock's elements is mettle and that of the goat is earth and there is an elemental coordination between both the elements, because mettle is a bi-product of earth. Hence an alliance (of marriage) and partnership between both signs can be forged and it will be successful also, as both can pull on together nicely. As the goat is a quadruped animal and cock has two legs, as a result of which marriage between the two partners will be incompatible. But, as far as partnership in business is concerned, both may pull on together.

12. Goat and Monkey

Monkey's element is mettle and goat's element is earth, and there is an affinity and congruity between both the elements, and both are complementary to each other also. But, the monkey is craftly cunning and mischievous and a trouble-shooter, where-as the goat is sober and composed by temperament, hence temperaments of both the animals are diametrically opposed to each other. So, both can not live together under one roof, nor will they remain happy. Persons of goat-sign will always remain tormented and troubled by the people of monkey-sign and, a spate of complaints will continue to surface.

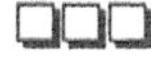

9. Monkey

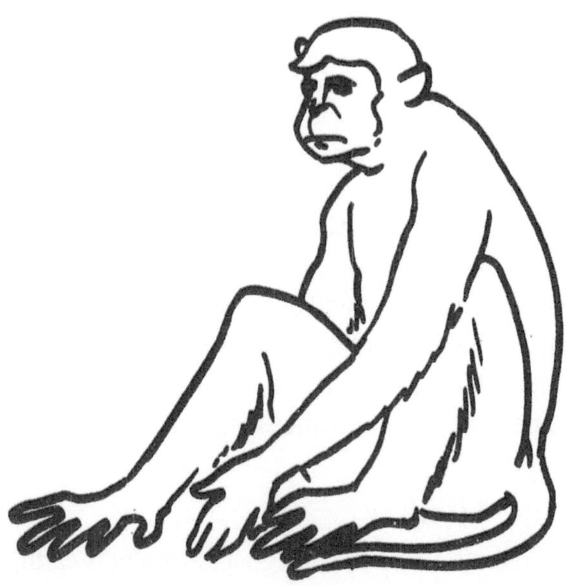

Natural Trait:– Trouble Shooter and Restive

Chinese Lunar Years						
02	February	1908	to	22	February	1909
20	February	1920	to	08	February	1921
06	February	1932	to	26	January	1933
25	January	1944	to	13	February	1945
12	February	1956	to	31	January	1957
29	January	1968	to	16	February	1969
16	February	1980	to	05	February	1981
04	February	1992	to	22	January	1993
22	January	2004	to	08	February	2005

Monkey

The 'Monkey' occupies ninth place in the Chinese zodiac circle and its element is mettle. Persons, born between 3.00 p.m. to 5.00 p.m. belong to Monkey-sign. It is situated between 217.5 and 247.5 degrees on the Chinese compass. It direction is situated between western and south-western (Vaayavya) directions.

The Monkey is an inqisitive animal and is firm in his belief, that is, it follows its plans himself. A persons born under the monkey sign is highly imaginative, intelligent and dedicated to the environment existing around him.

The animal is restive. It can not be preconceived which trick he would play with a person, that is it is unpredictable. To believe it is a totally unreliable advice and also helping other persons. The monkey is a totally unreliable animal.

Persons having monkey sign, are studious and love to participate in discussions and also arguments. Due their friendly and effective personality, they win the hearts of all people around them. They are capable of quickly finding solution to any problem and their solutions are wise. They are successful business persons, politicians and orators. But they are quite clever for their own gains.

Persons of monkey-sign are of vacillating nature, restive and can be courteous opportunists and can also forego their principles if they clash with their personal interests. At times, they can resort to even deceit and misappropriation in order to achieve their ends. Hence, such persons have very few friends due to their peculiar habits which stands to benefit them only. They are a bit lazy and idolent, hence seek resignation of their demanding and serious responsibilities. They concentrate on their petty problems and do not attend to more important problems of life. Monkey's can be quite easily misled, misguided.

Monkeys are past masters and experts in solving their problems. Monkey sign can befool even a strong animal like dragon, can deceive even a tiger and make the horse dance to its tune. That is to say that monkey is the cleverest of all the animals and can also pretended as if he is scared, but he is, actually, not afraid of anyone.

Hence, always keep in mind the said natural traits of the monkey, whenever making friends or enemies. Natural traits of the monkeys are also befooling, pilfering things and laughing at the distress of others.

The main weakness (rather a quality) of monkey sign people is that they manage to get their work accomplished, either by hook or cook, and when their objective has been achieved, they do not even follow the courtesy of thanking their friends and colleagues. It is neither their habit nor a trait to express gratitude, give thanks, nor preservation of culture and etiquetes. They can not digest and tolerate even an iota of disgrace either to themselves or the members or their clan. Moreover they will never forget if and when someone has insulted them, and they will not also rest until they have taken a revenge as they will take impact of insult of their heart.

1. Love Between Monkey and Mouse

If love affair between monkey and mouse sign matures into matrimony, it will make an excellent combination for a happy life. Mouse is intelligent and monkey is clever, hence when intelligence and cleverness join, it paves the way to an excellent and happy marital bliss. Element of mouse is water and that of monkey is mettle, and both have reciprocal affinity. Hence, if persons with monkey and mouse signs marry, or enter into business partnership, their bonds of love will be strong and lasting.

2. Monkey and Buffalo

Persons born under buffalo sign get attracted and effected by the those born under monkey sign, because the former requires latter's mischievousness and imaginative faculty, but both can not pull on together.

3. Monkey and Tiger make an incompatible pair

Tiger and monkey can not make a successful pair, because monkey is naughty and tiger dislikes monkey's naughtiness. Monkey is also unreliable and restive and these habits do not fit in tiger's mental frame, hence there is always animosity between both the signs.

4. Monkey and dragon's union fulfills high ambitions

Monkey's element is earth and that of dragon is earth, and mettle generates from earth itself, hence there is elemental affinity between both the signs. Hence due to elemental equality and affinity, it prepares the basis for fulfillment of aspirations and ambitions. Monkey's intellect and mischievousness and dragon's strength are complementary to each other; hence marriage and partnership between both creates an excellent atmosphere for a happy and prosperous life.

5. Monkey and Snake

Meeting of monkey and snake is actually an occasion for meeting of fire and earth elements, and there is also not natural enmity between the two. If both the signs could exhibit mutual understanding and sympathy, they can pull on amicably and lead a happy married life.

6. Monkey and Cat

Both can neither live nor pull on together.

7. Monkey and Horse

Element of horse is fire and that of monkey is metal, there is elemental equality between the two signs. Monkey remains attracted towards the horse, but the monkey has to remain dedicated to strength of the horse to sustain cordial relations.

8. Monkey and Goat

Monkey's element is metal and goat's element is earth. Both are complementary to each other and have natural affinity also. But monkey is highly clever and mischievous, whereas goat is sober, silent and simple, hence both have variable termperaments. So, both will not be able to live together under one roof, as persons with goat sign will remain tormented by those with monkey sign and thus a series of complaints will continue to surface.

9. Monkey and Monkey

There always exists attachment between one monkey and another as they belong to the same clan. All the monkeys move in a group and also help each other whenever there is some problem.

10. Monkey and Cock

Mettle is the common element of monkey and cock. Hence there is elemental affinity between them. Even then their approach is different from one another because cock is a simpleton and monkey is clever and trouble-shooter. Hence there is disparity between the approach and temperament.

11. Monkey and Dog

Element of monkey and dog is mettle and there is elemental equality between them. But monkey resorts to pilferage, whereas it is not the dog's habit. They are poles apart.

12. Monkey and Pig

Monkey's element is mettle and that of the pig is water, but the monkey is cleverer and a trouble shooter, but the pig is a pure hearted animal. Even if there is an ideological difference between them, owing to its accommodative sense, the pig can compromise and pull on also. He will be able to shoulder and sustain responsibility of home life, even if he has to tolerate the monkey's deplorable habits.

□□□

10. Cock

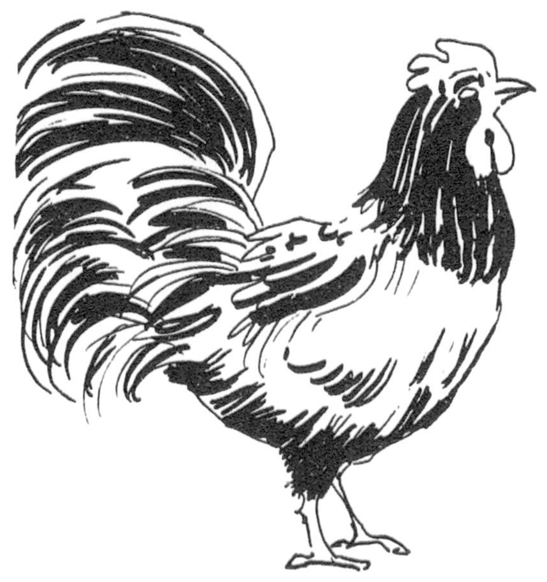

Natural Trait:– Talkative and Advice Voluntarily

Chinese Lunar Years						
22	January	1909	to	10	February	1910
08	February	1921	to	28	January	1922
26	January	1933	to	14	February	1934
13	February	1945	to	02	February	1946
31	January	1957	to	16	January	1958
17	February	1969	to	05	February	1970
05	February	1981	to	24	January	1982
23	January	1993	to	09	February	1994
09	February	2005	to	28	January	2006

Cock

The Vietnamese call the cock 'Chicken' and the Japanese call it a "Rooster".

Cock occupies tenth place in the Chinese zodiacal circle and its element is mettle. Persons, born between 5.00 p.m. and 7.00 p.m. have their sign as 'cock' and are called 'roosters' also. It has between 247.5 and 277.5 degrees in the Chinese compass. Its place falls under the western direction and can be located in the compass.

Persons of cock-sign are hard-working, affluent, resourceful and licentious. They pay full attention to even the minutest details in their work. They do not like disturbance, they love solitude and wish a secluded life. They are persons of indolent nature and keep harping on imaginary aspects, hence they generally do not succeed. They love to participate in discussions and arguments. They do not hesitate to speak out truth. They are restive, but are good organisers also. So they plan their programmes and activities well in advance. They take much interest in environmental and humanitarian activities. They serve people selflessly and feel whatever they are doing, that's perfectly in order. They consider themselves as 'heroes' and 'philosophers' and thus overrage themselves, because, in reality, they are not what they consider themselves to be.

Such natives are most suited to professions connected to publicity and media disciplines. They can also be good teachers. At times they show overconfidence due to which, their image gets tarnished . They are actually mad lovers and can go to any extent in love affairs. They have been seen to be successful in work relating to agriculture.

Persons of cock sign are well wishes of their clan. They eat one grain and throw the other one on the hind side so that the same could be consumed by other cocks.

Their old age is generally prosperous and comfortable. It is generally held that two persons of cock-sign can not live together peacefully under one roof. Despite a cock being a well wisher of his own clan, it will not hesitate to attack another cock when challenged or provoked.

1. Cock and Buffalo are excellent friends

According to the Chinese astrology cock and buffalo are highly intimate friends because both think alike. Buffalo's element is earth and that of cock is metal, and metal is a biproduct of earth. So, there is an element friendship between both the signs. Both the signs will mutually maintain love whether it is home, business or family life and tied in marital wedlock, they will mount bonds of love. Their animal life will forge ahead in mutual understanding for a long time.

2. Cock and Snake complement each other

According to Chinese belief, persons of cock and snake signs have common ways to act, think and conduct things. Snake's element is fire and that of cock is metal, and fire melts metal, hence persons of cock-sign are ever ready to sacrifice their life for the persons with snake sign. So (marital) wedlock between both signs is said to be an ideal one, because both the signs appreciate each other and ready to sacrifice for the sake of the other.

3. Cock and Mouse

There will be continuous and mutual arguments between persons of this sign, because mouse is a critic and cock indulges in making uncalled for and unproductive announcements, that is one views with the other and the vice versa. So there can not be any partnership between both the signs.

4. Cock and Tiger

It is quite difficult, if not impossible, for both the animals to pull on together. Hence whenever either of them wishes to establish partnership with the other, they should reciprocally weigh all the pros and cons thoroughly.

5. Cock and Dragon

There is a possibility of love-affairs between cock and dragon signs and, after their marriage, they become happy. After marriage the women generally gains dominance.

6. Cock and Cat

Due to inherent animosity between the cock and cat, they can not get along because persons of cat sign will never trust persons of cock sign, and cock-sign also does not repose its confidence on these with cat sign for the latter's tricky nature.

7. Cock and Horse

Cock's element is metal and that of the horse is fire and fire melts metal. So, there is elemental affinity and similarity between both the signs of these elements. But, horse is a powerful animal while the cock has weak will power. Hence if the cock remains dedicatedly sincere to the horse. They will make a useful and productive partnership.

8. Cock and Goat

Cock's element metal and goat's element is earth, and there is natural co-ordination and they are also complementary to each other, hence there may be a viable friendship, marriage and partnership between persons of these elements : But, the goat has four legs and the cock has only two legs. Hence they will make compatible marriage partners, but if they join hands in a partnership, it may work out to be a successful experience.

9. Cock and Monkey

Metal is the common element of both the animals and both may manage to pull on together. But the monkey and cock will have a variant approach between them. So, due to their inherent individual traits, they may find it difficult to pull on.

10. Cock and Cock

If sign of both the persons is identical the male cock can pull on with the female. Either they will fight with each other or kill themselves during the course of fighting.

11. Cock and Dog

Element of both of the cock and dog is metal and there is a natural friendship between both of them, but they are natural enemies also, and nobody knows when their suppressed feelings of enmity will arise. Moreover, nobody knows when they may get provoked and start fighting with each other. Hence a wedlock between both the signs is not said to be successful and productive.

12. Cock and Pig

Cock's element is metal but that of the pig is water and there is no elemental common factor between the signs and their mental approach is also not similar. So, their meeting and partnership is neither desirable nor even advisable.

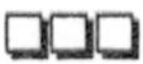

11. Dog

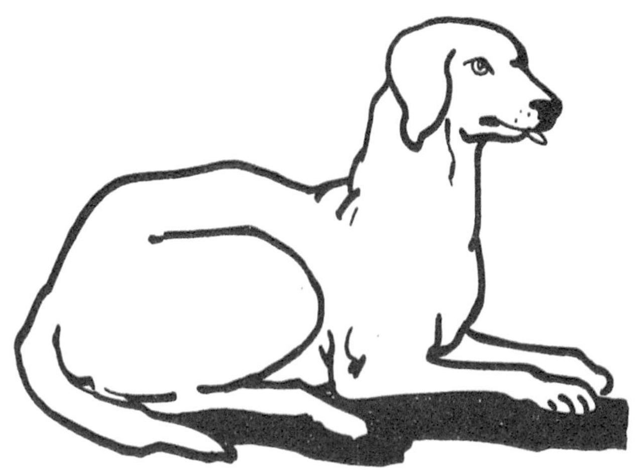

Natural Trait:– Faithful and Honest to its Master

Chinese Lunar Years						
10	February	1910	to	30	January	1911
28	February	1922	to	16	February	1923
14	February	1934	to	04	February	1935
02	February	1946	to	22	January	1947
16	February	1958	to	08	February	1959
06	February	1970	to	26	January	1971
25	January	1982	to	12	February	1983
10	February	1994	to	30	January	1995
29	January	2006	to	17	February	2007

Dog

Dog occupies eleventh place in Chinese zodiac circle. Its elements is metal. Persons, born between 5.00 p.m. and 7.00 a.m. have their element as metal. It is situated between 277.5 and 307.5 degrees on the Chinese compass. It is situated in the western direction.

Persons born under the dog sign are trust worthy, honest and strong-willed. They are frank and also the first persons to raise their voice to oppose, injustice and tyranny. They hate all the unlawful and unsustainable dealings. They consider themselves lucky when they have to help the needy, poor and the deserving. They listen to others opinion, but are also capable of convincing others . Though dog is not much of a social animal its nature is friendly. They do not like to participate in functions, instead they prefer to spend time with their friends. People born with dog sign are faithful and trust worthy but, if ever ill treated they will hardly forgive their tormentor.

Persons, having dog-sign, do not believe much in accumulating money. To meet their objective determinedly. Even if the dogs are cool-minded animals, they will never take rest, because they do not have any time to relax and rest. Even while they are relaxing or resting, their mind remains always active and engaged on some matter or the other. Persons of dog-sign find it rather difficult to make friendship with an unknown person but, once they be friend of a person, their relation of friendship stay forever.

These are courageous. If we take realistically, dog is the only animal who possesses all the qualities of nobility, in relation to twelve signs of 'Chi'. Their human traits are fidelity, loyalty, alert. There hardly are any other species of animals and humans who could match the excellence of dogs qualities, as they are never found wanting in the discharge of their duties. Dogs possess strong power and have also the capacity to foresee any impending danger. They never mistake while recognising their foes or friends. They never entertain nor tolerate anybody's interference in the field of their activity. They are champions in their own field, and if they determine to acquire anything will take rest only after they have attained their objective. They have firm belief in equality and relations of equal footing and whenever they feel their authority and rights are being intruded upon they will not hesitate to resort to fighting in order to preserve and protect their rights.

Persons having dog-sign are successful trade union leaders, religious preachers and authorities on religion, industrialists, editors, lawyers and distinguished orators. Their childhood passes in uncertainties, youth in struggle and service of other and in old age they have to shed tears. Persons of this sign who are born during the day time are more sober, calm and happy than those born during the night time.

1. Couple of Dog and Tiger forebodes excellent fortune

If dog and tiger sign persons are tied in a wedlock, it embellishes their fortune. Dog is an admirer of tiger and tiger is also an admirer of dog's fidelity and trust. Dog's element is earth and that of tiger is wood, and wood grows on the earth. So, the meeting of a woman having dog-sign and a man of tiger sign make a highly successful couple, because dog is female and tiger is male.

2. Pair of Dog and Horse remains stable upto the final stage

Marriage between dog and horse sign is always auspicious and their marriage remains stable even upto the end, because they make a happy and successful couple. If male's sign is horse then the dog-sign will always pay heed to the horse sign, and also understanding. Horse is ambitious and his progress pleases the dog. Hence both are reciprocally happy and satisfied with each other's progress. So, both are complementary to each other, that's why they are able to pull on together nicely.

3. Dog and Mouse

There is hardly any chance of pulling together and living congenially because both take pleasure in unnecessarily tormenting the other one.

4. Dog and Buffalo

Friendship between the dog and the buffalo is possible, if both the partners mutually trust each other and if they do so they can always attain heights of accomplishments.

5. Dog and Cat

Dog and cat can pull on together. But, since both are natural enemies, their animosity could be the basis of their feud, hence great caution is called for to forge an alliance between the two signs.

6. Dog and Dragon

Since, according to the Chinese belief, both the dragon and dog are each other's enemies, so any marriage and partnership between persons of these signs will be unmatching unproductive.

7. Dog and Snake

Meeting of the dog and snake is, in fact, a meeting of fire and metal elements, hence there is a natural friendship between both the signs. If there is mutual understanding and sympathy between the two, their meeting can be happy and fruitful.

8. Dog and Goat

Even if there exists element equality between the signs of both the animals, yet they can hardly pull on together, because they are natural enemies. Hence, it is difficult for them to live under one roof.

9. Dog and Monkey

Metal is the common element of both the dog and the monkey and they have elemental unity also. But their nature is oppose to each other. Monkey's nature is causing pilferage (theft) and dog is against any type of pilferage. So, there will always remain an ideological difference between the two. Hence, they will not be able to pull on together, despite having the same element.

10. Dog and Cock

Metal is the common element of both the dog and the cock, they have elemental friendship also, but there is also natural enmity between them. Nobody can foretell when such an enmity may erupt and result in a feud. So, their marriage is not recommended, due to the abovesaid factors.

11. Dog and Dog

Friendship between the two male persons of dog sign can be hardly productive and fruitful. If both the male persons belong to the same family or religion, it is in order, otherwise personal animosity and squabbling will continue to surface. But, it is also a fact the male dog-sign, and female dog-sign will continue to be fascinated each other, but such attraction will only be limited to satisfaction of sexual urge and will not lead to marital wedlock.

12. Dog and Pig

Dog's element is earth and that of the pig is water, and it is water that imparts production capability to the earth. If the woman is of dog-sign and man is of pig-sign, then their marriage will be successful and also pull on together nicely.

❑❑❑

12. Pig

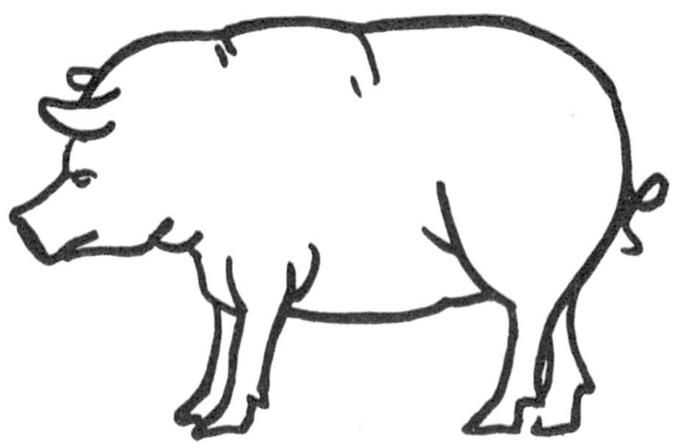

Natural Trait:– Pure Hearted, Simple and Upright (Honest)

Chinese Lunar Years						
30	January	1911	to	18	February	1912
16	February	1923	to	05	February	1924
04	February	1935	to	24	January	1936
22	January	1947	to	10	February	1948
08	February	1959	to	28	January	1960
27	January	1971	to	14	February	1972
13	February	1983	to	01	February	1984
31	January	1995	to	18	February	1996
18	February	2007	to	06	February	2008

Pig

The pig occupies twelfth in Chinese zodiac circle and its element is water. Persons borne between 9.00 p.m. and 11.00 p.m. are born under this sign. It occupies place between 307.5 and 337.5 degree on the Chinese compass.

Persons, whose zodiac sign is pig, are upright and pure hearted persons. They are cultured, compassionate, considerate, wise and capable of establishing peace due to their honesty and never tell lies. Due to their high sense of truthfulness they sometimes turn sceptical and suspicious. Since they rely and confide too much in others, they are be fooled and taken for a ride by people. They do not like depressed situations and spend up their force in recovering difference between two persons. They are truthful and have utmost faith in justice.

Persons of pig zodiac sign fully cooperate in establishing rule of law and order. They are jolly, at times, enjoy jokes or comments. They always aim at keeping others in good humour and entertaining them. Their power of self-confidence and character helps them to remove obstacle quickly that stand in the way to their progress. They are fortunate beings but, at the same time, are lazy and indolent also, In the matter of love, they are hypersensitive. They firmly believe in welcoming their guests. Women of this sign are always dedicated to their family and serve it. They consider it their pious duty to keep their husbands in a happy mind and look after their children.

Persons of pig-sign do not believe in finding faults, rather they analyse their own conduct and try to find out their own pitfalls and faults. This habit is the height of their gentle character. They set out clear goals for themselves and do not rest until they have achieved their targeted objectives, due to their strong determination. But they analyse all factors minutely and also the circumstances around them, hence due to this reason, their achievements get delayed and, at times, it looks as if they have deviated from their path.

Persons of this sign have very fewer friends in life. But once they forge friendship with any person, they continue to sustain this friendship throughout life. They also do not bother whether their friends reciprocate their friendly gesture or not, that's why their love-affair is also one-sided, as they do not bother whether their beloved responds to their sincere love in the same vein or not. Like the dog, they also believe in picking up feuds. Though they are slow in action, yet they firmly proceed towards their targeted aim, even if at a snails space species and ultimately achieve their objective. They are capable of displaying and proving their capability and efficiency in the field of art, painting, music, poetry, writing etc. as they succeed more in such fields than other fields. The most agonising irony of their fate is that they are always deceived in love. Other persons, will have sympathy for them, but their relatives and friends will always ditch them.

1. Pig and Cat will Pull on together

As per Chinese beliefs marriage between pig and cat signs continues without any obstacle and both partners will be ever ready for sacrifice. Their marriage will be an ideal one and business partnership will also be ideal and successful.

2. Pig and Mouse

Since element of both the signs is water, their marriage, business and partnership will last lifelong and they will have faith in each other, and both will also suddenly get good objects.

3. Pig and Buffalo

If pig and buffalo are tied in a wedlock, their married life will be an ideal one.

4. Pig and Tiger

Persons of pig sign will feel scared of the tiger sign and this will be an unpendimental factors in their marriage.

5. Pig and Dragon

Meeting between persons of both the signs is possible and both can pull on also. But persons of pig sign have to make greater sacrifices.

6. Pig and Snake

If a person of snake sign marries a member of opposite sex of the pig sign, then snake will dominate over the selfless and upright Pig. If male sign is snake, he will continue to reprimand his wife for her mistakes, and ladies of Pig-sign will continue to bear the rebukes like dedicated wives so that family does not get disturbed. But if a marriage takes place, it will not be an ideal marriage, due to their divergent elements. Element of snake is fire and that of pig is water, and both have elemental variables.

7. Pig and Horse

Pig's dominant element is water and that of the horse is fire and their is mutual enmity between the two elements. Moreover horse is a fast animal, whereas, pig is innocent and simple. There are also ideological disparities between them apart from variation in speed of activity–the horse is a fast moving animal and pig is painfully slow. Hence persons of both the signs will not make a matching couple, and can not live in amity under one roof.

8. Pig and Goat

Extent and depth of love between the pig and goat is indescribable in words. Sensitive goat feels obliged to have a partner in the form of pig's selfless and pure love. Goat's element is earth, whereas that of pig is water and as water emerges from the earth, so it imparts in earth, the capacity to produce. Hence when pig and goat signs combine in a wedlock, they both give birth to excellent progeny. Both will feel happy when either of them do and thing for the other partner. Hence marriage, partnership and love affair between the pig and goat signs will remain happy and sustainable.

9. Pig and Monkey

Monkey's dominant element is metal while pig's dominant element is water. The monkey is naughty and mischievous and the pig is pure and simple animal. Through there exists elemental disparity between the sign yet pig will manage to compromise. So, in order to discharge all family obligations, it will tolerate even monkey's sign mischief.

10. Pig and Cock

There is no elemental parity between both the signs, because pig's element is water, while that of the cock is metal, and their line of thinking is also opposite. Hence, their mutual marriage and partnership is not advisable.

11. Pig and Dog

Dog's element is earth and that the dog is water, and water saturate earth to enable it to produce various products. If woman's sign is dog and that of man is pig, then their marriage will be successful and they will also be able to pull on together for the purpose of discharging their worldly obligations.

12. Pig and Pig

Combination of pig and pig is like a heaven on earth, because both have an urge to lie for the benefit and welfare of each other, and will also remain committed to each other. Both have patience and love between them which is also selfless. It hardly matters which of the two partners has its signs as pig, but it is the fact that both will live in perfect cooperation, and spend their life nicely by discharging their respective duties. In the foregoing pages details of 12 Chinese signs of their zodiac circle have been mentioned and the Chinese lunar years ascribed to a particular sign, its characteristic individual traits and ancient signs relations and impact in combination with other animal signs have also been detailed.

PART–2
I-Ching

6
Introduction to I-CHING

Yen and yang are nature's two energy flowing channels which bring about changes in the universe and it has got a vast range. Reference to I-Ching appears in an ancient Chinese writer's (Fu Hsi) legendary treatise, entitled-I-Ching or book of changes and this book is a gift for the human civilization. In the said book, a new system of predicitions has been evolved and the system has been explained by establishing coordination between three horizontal unbroken and three broken transverse lines in an octogonal trigram. Legend has it that a golden yellow dragon emerged from Logave river, who blessed Fu Hsi with Chi power of writing. Fu Hsi was China's emperor. It is not possible to tell the exact date of writing this Book, but it is certain the said Book existed and popularised before 1100 B.C.

ली (Li)	अग्नि तत्व (fire)
कुन (K'un)	पृथ्वी तत्व (earth)
टुई (Tui)	दलदल (marsh)
चाईन (Ch'ien)	स्वर्ग (heaven)
कान (K'an)	जल तत्व (water)
केन (Ken)	पर्वत (mountain)
चेन (Chen)	विद्युत (thunder)
सन (Sun)	वायु तत्व (wind)

It is traditionally believed that Yen and Yang (energies) flow in a straight line. In I-Ching, Yen is represented by a broken line while Yang is represented by an unbroken transverse line. When three lines of Yen and Yang are positioned over each other, either trigram are formed, and each trigram represents and element each-this is explained as under:-

Two sets of trigram are made, this is 64 diagram/forms are made by congoursing six lines except lines of Yang and Yen. Which in Chinese parlance is called a 'Hexagram'. In I-Ching a result is mentioned in each of the hexagrams, and such results pertain to an individual's internal natural strength. Character and natural tracts or elements. Those results were formulated by C hina's emperor Keng Wen who ruled China in 1160 B.C. After his death is son introduced certain amendments to it. Yen, after 10 years China's renowned scholars, Confucious, carried out same specific experiment which were also aded to the Hexagram, so, traditional modifications were inducted in these Hexagrams.

In each Hexagram coordination between Yen and Yang has been indicated and also that conditions keep on changing every second in this universe and, thus, such change cast impact impact on each individual's life. All such beliefs are alluded to Chinese 'Taorgin' where an attempt has been made to look into deep mysteries and changing phenomenon. Feng Shui is a medium through which we try to comprehend principles of Tao, and environments.

7
Method to understand a Hexagram

Before we try to understand Feng Shui science, it is necessary to know what it meant by the term 'Hexagram', that it pertains to, what mystery lies behind it, how it can be studied, what is its utility and how and in which way is it related to I-Ching?

'Hex' means Six, and Hexagram means a figure/diagram having six angles. It has six parallel lines. It is formed by conjunction of two diagrams.

There are three parallel lines in a trigram, these lines are complete/ unbroken and also broken. Three complete or three broken lines when formed together, form eight, trigrams of different formations, depending on variable situations. The following diagrams will explain what I wish to convey and explain.

ATTRIBUTES OF TRIGRAMS

Trigram	Name	Attribute
☰	**Ch'ien** FATHER	**CREATIVE** Strong/Head/Horse Dark Red/ Heaven
☳	**Chen** FIRST SON	**THE AROUSING** Movement/Thunder Dragon/Inciting Foot
☵	**K'an** SECOND SON	**ABYSMAL** Peril/Danger/Water The Pit/Pig/Ear
☶	**Ken** THIRD SON	**KEEPING STILL** Mountain/Repose/Hand Fingers/Dog

ATTRIBUTES OF TRIGRAMS

Trigram	Name	Attribute
☷	**K'un** MOTHER	**RECEPTIVE** Belly/Cow-Mare Form/Yielding/Earth
☴	**Sun** FIRST DAUGHTER	**GENTLE** Wood-Wind/Cock Penetration/Thighs
☲	**Li** SECOND DAUGHTER	**CLINGING** Pleasant/Brightness/Eye yellow/Clarity/Flame/Fire
☱	**Tui** THIRD DAUGHTER	**JOYFUL** Lake/Marsh/Mouth Green-Blue/Sheep/Pleasurable

When both the above referred trigram are joined, it constitutes a Hexagram. When 8x8 different trigram are formed /multiplied, it given us 64 Hexagrams.

These 64 Hexagrams represent human's soul and character which are laid open by power and elements from nature. Each lines used in these Hexagrams discloses one's fortune or misfortune. Aspirant's inquisitive posers can also be replied through these hexagons, and some of the questions could be personal or also social read carefully the heading on card no. 56 of the hexagram, you will see its heading is 'Travelling Stranger'. The upper trigram denotes fire, shine and beauty and the lower trigram is indicative of mountain.

Movable lines no. 6 and 9 indicate a separate divine meaning which should be determined and understood from the result mentioned on the back side of the card. There are two moveable lines at figure no. 56 of the hexagram. Line no. 6 is situated at the second place and moveable line no. 9 from where Yang energy emanates, is situated at the fourth place. Posting of line. no. 6 at the sixth place is an indication that the subject traveller enjoys all the facilities with regard to comfortable stay, servants, pageantry, and means of livelihood to sustain life-in fact, all these aspects point out to excellent fortune.

Posting of Line no. 6 at fourth place denotes that the traveller is living in a rest house and has an axe and other means of livelihood, and he is an intelligent person to. This movable line also indicates that circumstances are changing, and also that more changes are also possible.

A movable line indicates flow and change. Hence when a person's future has already been predicted, the movable will denote the changed situations subsequent to the preliminary forecast. Hence the movable line will indicate the changes that are due to take up, after one's future has already been predicted. Such post Prediction changes are indicated through Yen line (**X**) and thus the predictions are at variance with what had already been predicted. But and Yen line indicates negative results. If two movable lines (in Hexagon) are changed to two immovable lines, we will obtain the following hexagon, No -18.

	Hexagon 56	**Changed**	**Hexagon 18**	
	7 ▬▬▬	Yang Line	▬▬▬	
LI	8 ▬ ▬	Yin Line	▬ ▬	Ken
	9 ▬O▬	Yin Line	▬ ▬	
	7 ▬▬▬	Yang Line	▬▬▬	
Ken	6 ▬X▬	Yang Line	▬▬▬	Sun
	8 ▬ ▬	Yin Line	▬ ▬	

As is apparent from the above description a new hexagon is constructed with the help of Ken and Sun which aggregates to numerical number 18 and the nomeaclature of this hexagon is Ku and the implied import of this hexagon is 'Arresting Decay'. They upper trigram represents a mountain which denotes 'Arresting Progress', while the lower trigram represents wood and wind elements, meaning, by turning over this card of the hexagram you will obtain the following predictive result which is noted in the back side of the hexagon.

"Ku indicates high activity and success. The work is not an easy one it takes wading and penetrating through a waterfall so as to reach the other end. So, the persons who wishes to plunge into any job, should take into consideration the difficulties and disparities involved before he starts. He should than take up the work after three days, after fully examining the complications and problems he may have to face."

Hence hexagon Nos. 56 and 18 imply that questioner's failure or success is dependent on change. He should also be reasonably cautioned and that he is heading towards those difficult situations about which he himself knows very little; because the forthcoming changes could be auspicious ominous even, and it can not be said with any amount of certainty what is in store for him or what will be the outcome of his efforts. So, he should be mentally prepared for either of the results.

Small dots will be noticed on the back side of Hexagon No. 64 which will consist of one or two lines. These are highly significant dots that indicate the main line which control and administers the hexagon, If Yang line is in an unbroken and complete (–) stage and if it is positioned in the first, third and fifth places, it will impart excellent and favourable results. But, when the Yen line is broken (– –) and incomplete and is also posted in the second, fourth and sixth places, it is an auspicious sign. While counting the numerical number, one should start counting from below and proceed upwards.

I went to China's capital Peking, in 1990, and also visited countries like Hongkong, Bangkok, Singapore, Makau. There I saw many I-Ching foretellers. They were sitting under shades of trees in the open or under canopies. I also stood in their future. It was, indeed, a pleasant experience. World of 'I-Ching is full of surprises and scintillating experiences and is quite popular in Central Asia and Europe. It is revealed through dices, coins and playing cards. Following relevant details of each method would be of interest to the readers.

1. Prediction through Dices

In India also, predictions are made by using dices in 'Ramal Science' similarly. I saw dices, made out of ivory. They have eight ivory dices where upon entire I-Ching has been etched. These dices are kept in beautiful vertical containers. The foreteller chants mantras, shakes all the containers and drops them on a silver plate upon which picture of deity of fortune has been painted. The aspirants touches a dices out of the eight dices. Then the forletter chants the mantra's again and spreads the dices on the golden plate. The diagram of the hexagon, as shown above, is actually indicative of the questioner's luck.

2. Prediction through Coins

Coins, made out of eight metals, are available in China and diagrams of all the 64 hexagrams are etched on these coins. Three aspirants, while speaking 'Manibhadra Hoon Phatt' mantra's places up a coin and the picture of a diagram, etched the coin, denotes luck or fortune of the aspirant. There also many others methods in vogue for using the coins so as to foretell future of an aspirant.

A specific method to foretell by using coins

Entire I-Ching can be seen to have been elected on three main coins which are used in China for predicting future. You may take three coins of any side each coin has a Head' (Front side) and 'Tail' (Back side). When the term 'Head' is used, it notes three complete unbroken (▬)Yang lines, while the back portion denotes two incomplete broken(▬ ▬)

Yen lines. All the three coins are put on the palm, first is closed and shaken or even the three coins be put in a cup, its mouth covered by a hand, and then the cup is shaken (—) one can use either of the methods according to availability and convenience. Then drop the coins three lines and jot down the resultant details on a piece of paper. It should be kept in mind that the 'Head' indicates 3 complete lines and the 'Tail' indicates 2 broken lines. Now the following figurations can emerge, viz

(A) Three 'Tail sides'
(2+2+2) = 6 = —X— that is movable Yin Line

(B) Two 'Tails' and one 'Head'
(2+2+3) = 7 = — Immovable Yang Line

(C) Two 'Head' and one 'Tail'
(3+3+2) = 8 = — — Immovable Yin Line

(D) Three 'Heads'
(3+3+3) = 9 — Movable Yang Line

When the coins are thrown, one of the above mentioned results or figurations are arrived at. One Toss of coins results in formation of a trigram. It may be borne in mind that when the three coins are 'tossed' for the first time, it constitutes (forms) lower line of the trigram, and the second toss results in formation of the upper line. This is how six tosses of coins, results in formation of six lines of the hexagon.

It should also be kept in mind that line Nos. 6 and 9 are called movable lines. Hence coins are tossed thrice the results of the 'Tail-side' would be 2+2+2 = 6 and three tosses of the coins resulting in 'Head-side' will devote a total of 9 (3+3+3 = 9), which means that figure '6' denotes movable Yin energy while the figure '9' denotes immovable Yang energy.

Movable line is the leading basis for divine predictions and all the results are mentioned in the head side of 64 hexagon cards.

Here, some of the examples are being given which spell out the importance of Yin and Yang lines, consequently observed after tossing the coins.

1. **First Toss:** 3+2+3 = 8, immovable Yin lines. — —
   that is Head + Tail and Head.
2. **Second Toss:** 2+2+2 = 6, mobile Yin lines. —X—
   that is Head + Head.
3. **Third Toss :** 2+3+2 = 7, immovable Yang lines, ——
   that is Tail + Head-Tail.
4. **Fourth Toss:** 3+3+3 = 9, mobile Yang line ——
   Head + Head + Head

5. **Fifth Toss:–** 3+2+3 = 8, immovable Yen line ▬ ▬
Head + Tail + Head.
6. **Sixth Toss :–** 2+3+2 = 7, immovable Yang line ▬▬▬
by tossing the coins for six times, following hexagrams are constituted, viz.
7. Yang line ▬▬▬
8. Yen line ▬ ▬
9. Mobile Yang line ▬▬▬
10. Yang line ▬▬▬
11. Mobile Yen line ▬X▬
12. Yen line ▬ ▬

When this hexagon is compared with 'table of the Hexagon". You will find that the lower trigram is 'Ken' and the upper one is 'Li'. According to this chart when we compare trigram 'Ken' with 'Li' we obtain figure '56' of the Hexagon and name of the Hexagon will be 'L'.

3. Prediction through Playing cards

These days playing cards in I-Ching, are also used in Europe and central Asia where some people call 'I-Ching' and 'EA CHING". A left is supplied with the I-Ching cards where in reductions have been briefly explained. Following are printed on the playing cards-

(a) Name of the Hexagram in Chinese.
(b) Six parallel lines of the Hexagram
(These lines are read from down upwards)
(c) Several numbers of the Hexagram
(d) Name of the Hexagram in English
(e) Name of the Trigram related in Hexagram
(f) Ingredients relating to a Trigram.

Prediction is divided into two parts and is written on the back side of the cards. One on the upper part and other on the lower part. One on the upper part the meaning of the hexagon and its mystical meaning are written which are meant for a welfare of the aspirants. On the lower portion individual prediction is written. Such predictions are based upon each parallel lines. These lines are two-

1. unrboken and 2. broken

Unbroken line

An unbroken lines is called 'Line No. 9' which is also a movable line and it denotes Yang energy. It is marked by affixing 'O' sign which is represented by a straight line, like –O–. The line which is not mobile is called by the code name '7'. Which actually is a Yang line and is denoted by a straight line as ▬▬▬

Broken line

It is a movable line which is denoted by numerical number '6' which represents Yen energy. It is indicated by inserting the sign 'X' in between the broken lines as ▬▬X ▬▬A line, which is not a movable line, is indicated by a broken line that represents yen line. This line is called by numerical number "8".

Now it is well clear that in a code language Yen line is called "6" and "8" and the Yang line "7" and "9". Such points must always be borne in mind while studying the hexagons.

Modification chart for the Hexagons

UPPER TRIGRAM	Ch'ien ☰	Chên ☳	K'an ☵	Kên ☶	K'un ☷	Sun ☴	Li ☲	Tui ☱
LOWER TRIGRAM	1	2	3	4	5	6	7	8
Ch'ien 1 ☰	1	34	5	26	11	9	14	43
Chên 2 ☳	25	51	3	27	24	42	21	17
K'an 3 ☵	6	40	29	4	7	59	64	47
Kên 4 ☶	33	62	39	52	15	53	56	31
K'un 5 ☷	12	16	8	23	2	20	35	45
Sun 6 ☴	44	32	48	18	46	57	50	28
Li 7 ☲	13	55	63	22	36	37	30	49
Tui 8 ☱	10	54	60	41	19	61	38	58

Introduction to 1 to 64 Hexagrams

8 pi	7 sze	6 sung	5 hsû	4 măng	3 kun	2 khwån	1 khien
16 yü	15 khien	14 tâ yû	13 thung zăn	12 phi	11 thâi	10 li	9 hsiâo khû
24 fù	23 po	22 pi	21 shih ho	20 kwân	19 lin	18 kù	17 sui
32 häng	31 hsien	30 li	29 khan	28 tâ kwo	27 i	26 tâ khû	25 wû wang
40 kiah	39 kien	38 khwei	37 kià zan	36 ming I	35 zin	34 tâ kwang	33 thun
48 zing	47 khwân	46 shâng	45 zhui	44 kâu	43 kwâi	42 yi	41 sun
56 jü	55 fâng	54 kwei mei	53 kien	52 kăn	51 kăn	50 ting	49 ko
64 wei zi	63 ki zi	62 hsiâo kwo	61 kung fû	60 kieh	59 hwân	58 tui	57 sun

8
Names And Meanings of 64 Hexagrams

	Chinese Name	Hindi Prounciation	Meaning
1.	Ch'ien	चैन	Origin
2.	K'un	कुन	Success
3.	Chun	चुन	Birth pangs
4.	Meng	मैंग	Naughty and trouble shooter
5.	HSU	हसु	Patience
6.	Sung	सुंग	Argument
7.	Shen	शीह	Army
8.	Pi	पीह्	Organization
9.	H Sie ch'u	हुसिया'चु	Low Capability
10.	Chun	चुन	Birth pangs
11.	T'ai	ताई	Philanthropy
12.	P'i	पी	Hindrance
13.	T'ungJen	तुंग जेन	Associate, Friend
14.	Ta Yu	तायू	Multiple Rights
15.	Ch'ien	चैन	Humidity
16.	Yu	यू	Courage, Agility
17.	Sui	सुई	Approach upto a Compromise

18.	Ku	कु	Degradation.
19.	Len	लिन	Degradation.
20.	Kuan	कुआन	Text, Examination
21.	Shin Ho	शिन हो	Beating, Thrashing
22.	Pe	पी	Worth, Worshipping
23.	Po	पौ	Kind, Peeling
24.	Fu	फू	Return
25.	Wu Wang	वू वेंग	Honesty
26.	Ta ch'u	टा-चू	Great Power-Worth
27.	I	आई	Soon after, Taking Care
28.	Ta Kuo	टा कुओ	Great Experience
29.	K'an	कान	Deep Water
30.	Li	ली	Luster, Glamour
31.	Hsien	हसैन	Welcome, Reception.
32.	Heng	हेंग	Continuous
33.	Tun	टुन	Hiding
34.	Ta chuang	टा चुन्ग	Great Power
35.	Chin	चिन	Advance
36.	MingI	मिंग ई	Opaqueness, Unclear
37.	Chia Jen	चेन जेन	Fairly
38.	K'uei	कुई	Opposition
39.	Chien	चैन	Problem, Calamity
40.	HSien	हेसीह	Release, Freedom
41.	Sun	सन	Better Lines
42.	I	आई	Progress
43.	Kuai	कुऐं	New Games
44.	Kou	कोउ	Meeting, Joining
45.	T S'ui	ट्सुई	Together, Accumulate
46.	Sheng	सेंग	To Surge Ahead
47.	K'un	कुन	All Around
48.,	Ching	चिंग	The Best

49.	Ko	को	Change
50.	Ting	टिंग	Cauldren
51.	Chen	चेन	Shock, Push, Jerk
52.	Ken	केन	Rest, Relaxation
53.	Chien	चेन	Slow Progress
54.	Kuei Mei	कुई मै	Happiness
55.	Feng	फेंग	Progress
56.	Lu	लू	Joining, Travel
57.	Sun	सन	Civility, Goodness
58.	Tui	टुई	Mirth, Happiness
59.	Huan	हुआन	To Scatter, Spread
60.	Chieh	चैह	Limit, Boundary
61.	Chung Fu	चुंग फु	Internal Confidence
62.	Hsia o Kuo	हेसियौ कुओ	Minor Problem
63.	Chi-Chi	ची ची	Finalised, Completed
64.	Wei-chi	वेई ची	Not Yet Done Completely

Brief Description and Forecasting To each of the Hexagrams

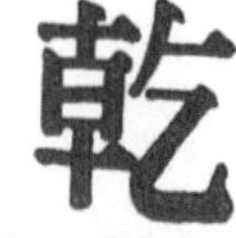

1. Chien

(Origin)–It is a hexagram consisting of 6 complete (unbroken) lines which are Yang lines. Since it is indicative of origin it had the nomenclature 'Chien' Trigram by which it is meant that it is a sign or symbol of all those objects which originate. The six lines shown, here represent strength and authority. The Chinese believe that. 'Chi'en Hexagram' develops and propels an object in the right way.

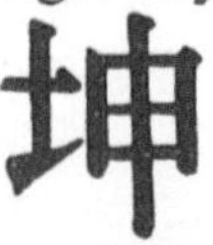

2. K'un

(Stands for Success) – This hexagon consists of six broken lines, hence, its nomenclature as 'K'ien. It stands for success. This trigram represents a peaceful and happy personality. It also indicates to a sober temperament, excellent health and strength. It also denotes the shape of a horse.

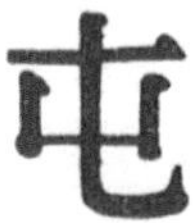

3. Chun

(It denotes Birth-Pang)—This Trigram is constituted like this --- first line is broken, the second is unbroken (complete), fourth and fifth lines are again broken lines, while the last (sixth) line is unbroken. This Trigram is considered water and electricity, forewarns a person that he must be cautious before he undertakes any new work/job, a symbol of danger and hallucination and guides one to minutely weigh the pros and cons of every work he is likely to undertake. It seeks help of noble persons who are able to guide and advise properly. Though you are sure to win ultimately yet caution is necessary.

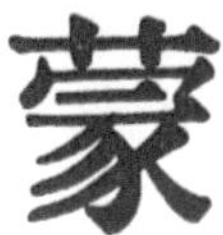

4. Meng

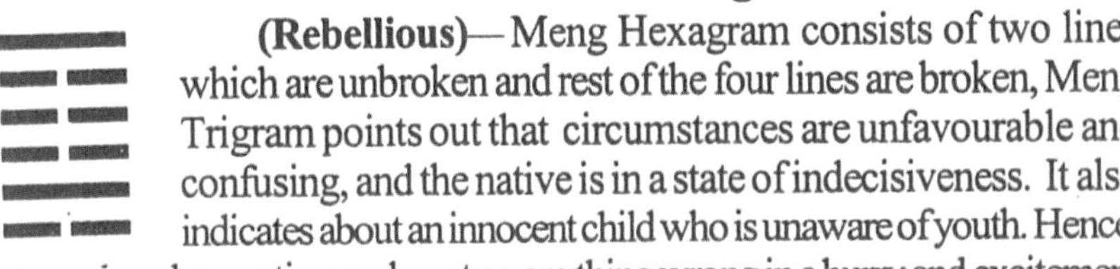

(Rebellious)— Meng Hexagram consists of two lines which are unbroken and rest of the four lines are broken, Meng Trigram points out that circumstances are unfavourable and confusing, and the native is in a state of indecisiveness. It also indicates about an innocent child who is unaware of youth. Hence, you need not lose patience, do not go anything wrong in a hurry and excitement or (provocation). If you can be patient, you will achieve success.

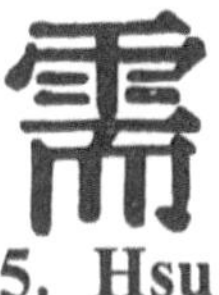

5. Hsu

Hsu hexagram stands for patience. It is a mixture of Ch'ien and K'an, apart from being a combination of water element and heaven. It is such a hexagram which given the impression as if clouds are rising from the earth. Even if the clouds and the earth look separate, there is interrelation between them --- as body and feelings look totally apart, even as there is correlation between them. Here the upper most line and third line are broken, while the other four are unbroken. This hexagram indicates and guides us that problem is lying ahead: hence minutely study the situation and environs all around and take recourse to patience while solving your problems.

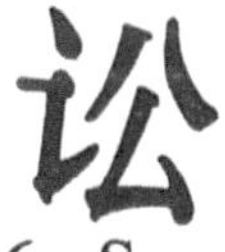

6. Sung

(Conflict)— This hexagon denotes conflict and the Trigram is a mix up of Ch'ien and K'an. It is also indicative of heaven and water (elements). It consists of four unbroken and two broken lines. It is also totally opposite to Hsu. It indicates that hard work is necessary for attaining success. Three upper protruding lines of the hexagram denote intellect and capacity to take the correct decision, whereas the lower lines are an indication of danger and wind. One need not feel depressed, and surge towards your goal with utmost caution.

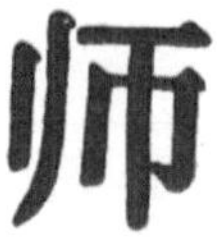

7. Shih

(Army)— This is known as the hexagram of Army and the Trigram is a combination of Kun and K'an. It is also a combination of earth and water elements. It consists of one unbroken and five broken lines, which indicate the strong persons know fully well how to discharge their duties for the welfare of the general public, and do not care at all for their selfish motives. This also points out that great achievements can be accomplished through mutual cooperation and understanding.

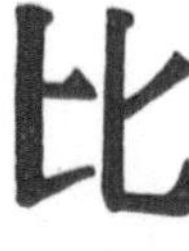

8. Pi

(Unity)___ This hexagram is called a hexagram of unit. It is a combination of K'an and K'un, and elements water and earth. In the Trigram there is only one unbroken line, while the other five lines are broken lines. It is absolutely reverse of 'Shih'. It denotes that danger exists in the lower portion, while the upper portion is comparatively safe and peaceful. It also indicates that if people work with mutual cooperation, they can attain success. If at all, any problem emerges, try to ward of the same at the earliest. It hardly matters whether you are wrong or right, even then seek counsel from other people and then start working.

小畜

9. Hsiao CH'U

(Low Capability/Ability)___ This is known as a Hexagram of "low capability". It is a combination of Ch'ien and Sun, and also of wind and heaven, While looking at the trigram one feels that clouds are hovering in the sky and there seem hardly any possibility of rainfall, though torrential rains may be notices enroute. It all indicates that a persons must be prepared to face all the impending probabilities. Moreover, one should have strong will-power, though one should look cheerful and unnerved outwardly. Other people might think that you are ready for a compromise, but inwardly you should forge ahead to accomplish your setout goal.

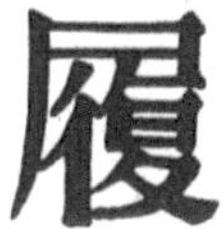

10. Li

(Tread Carefully)—This hexagon is a combined form of Chi'en and Tui which represent heaven and marsh. It is totally at variance with "Hsiav Ch'ug"" Hexagram and Trigram. It has no broken line and six unbroken lines. This sign is indicative of an organised society and milestone of formulation. It also warns against high ambition. This emblem represents honesty, capability and hard work, and also imparts success, provided the aspirant treads his path with great caution and care.

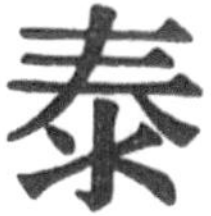

11. T' ai

(Benevolence and Philanthrophy)—It is called a "Hexagon of philanthropy and benevolence". The Trigram has three broken lines on its upper portion and three unbroken lines on its lower portion. It is conglomeration of K'un and Ch'ien and also of water element and heaven. It is a positive emblem. Which stands for love and tranquillity and also indicates existence of strong bonds of love between a man and a woman. This emblem also denotes strength, contemplative intelligence, determination, patience and perseverance. Combination of all the said traits helps one to achieve his goal, attain success and strengthen his will power.

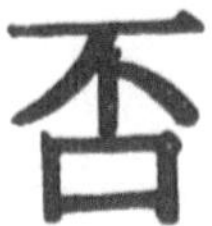

12. Pi

(Obstruction)— It is known as a "Hexagram of obstruction". It is a combination of Chi'en and Ku'n. Which also includes combination of heaven and earth. It is totally opposite to Tai, as it contains three unbroken lines on the upper portion and three broken lines on the lower portion. Here positive and negative energies will remain in continual confrontation, and nobody can foretell which of the two will dominate. It is said that this emblem resembles sandy earth, whose ever particle remains segregated. Hence it is an uphill task to establish coordination among the segregated particles. So, one has to have extreme patience and a strong will-power to bring the circumstances under control.

同人

13. T' ung Jen

(Companion)—It is called a "Hexagram of Companion". It is a combination 'Chi'en and Li and also of heaven and fire. The trigram has one broken line and five unbroken lines. It is a sign of positivity. So, all the persons, desirous of achieving their goal, should work in mutual coordination and with noble thinking. They should also arrive at collective decisions and also repose confidence mutually between one and another.

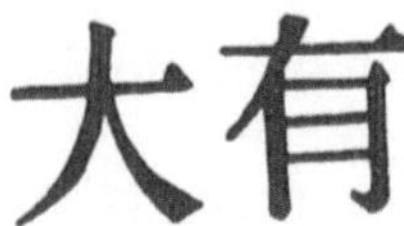

14. Ta Yu

(Multiple Possessions)—Tayu is called a 'Hexagram of multiple possessions'. It is a combination of 'Li' and 'Ch'ien and also heaven and fire elemment. As it has one broken line and five unbroken lines', it is totally at variance with 'Tang Jen' Trigram. It represents strength and courage, and also multiple possessions. The upper segment of the Trigram indicates obstruction and oddity (clumsiness and ugliness). Whereas the lines in the lower segment of the Trigram encourages noble and virtuous elements that means patiently listen to opinions of others. The nature then finds out a viable solution. Caution will pave the way for solution. Hence never act in undue hurry nor even change your standpoint every now-and then.

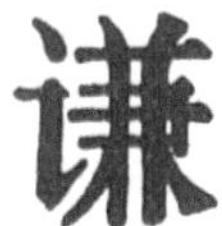

15. CH'ien

(Humility and Modesty) ____ Ch'ien is known as a "hexagram of modesty and humility". It is a combination of earth and mountain. It is also a conglomeration of K'un and Ken. It has one unbroken line, while the rest of five lines are broken. If you have authority then this symbol is indicative of importance of other people. But be cautious that your plans are meant for (the benefit of) others. So, give importance to others views so that they (people) respect you. And, if people give you respect, accept the same with humility and modesty.

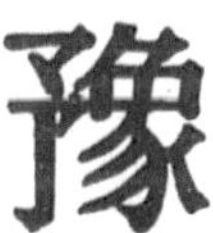

16. Yii

(Enthusiasm)—It is called a hexagon of Enthusiasm, It is a combination of 'Chien' and 'Kun' and also fire (electricity) and earth elements. Since it has only one unbroken line and five broken lines, it is totally opposite to 'Chien'. The Trigram indicates that success is in the offing. Its position lies in-between the positions of mother and her eldest son. Who does not show concern or agree with his mother's advice, but has a compromising approach also, such an approach is helpful in finding a solution to the problem. Compromise is an essential attribute that enables persons of forge ahead with confidence, understanding and zeal.

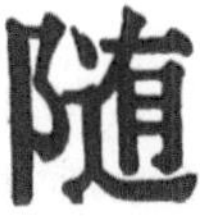

17. Sui

(Approach for a compromise or agreement)— This Hexagram stands for "a compromising approach" to reach an combination of thundering sound of clouds and march. This Trigram consists of one broken line at the top, followed by two unbroken fines in the middle, then there are two broken lines and an unbroken line at the end. 'Tui' Trigram denotes a tranquil nature while 'Chien' is active and powerful . Sui Hexagram is indicative of rainfall due to thunder of clouds. Rain converts marsh and mud into water, so that the stuck up and blocked work can get rid of obstacles, if others counselling is accepted. It also indicates that one will get a new thing so as to replace the old one.

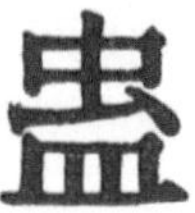

18. Ku

(Decay, Degradation)—It is called a "hexagon of decay." It is a combination of 'Ken; and 'Sun' which is indicative of mountain and wind. Its first line is unbroken, second and third line broken, fourth and fifth unbroken and last one is again broken. Hence, it is totally opposite to 'Sun' where there are three lines broken and three lines unbroken. This hexagram points out that we are passing good and bad phases. This emblem also indicates birth pang. It has been hard that where the boundaries of heaven end, the boundaries of hell emerge. When mystery of pain reach their final stage, thereafter one can hope to have favourable phase. If some new work is initiated, remember God and you will get help from somewhere.

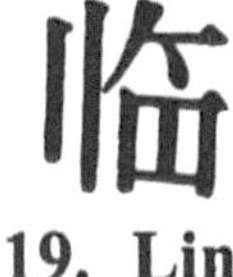

19. Lin

(Near Success)—This Hexagram is also known as that of a "Near Success". Its Trigram is a combination of 'K'un' and 'Dui' and also of earth element and swamp first four lines of this Trigram are broken, while the last two are unbroken. This Hexagram is indicative of productivity and courage. Earth element, with the help of mud, swamp and water helps towards productivity. It also indicates that the present time is meant for advice and experience of others to carry on partnership and, if it is done, one will feel success waiting at his doorsteps.

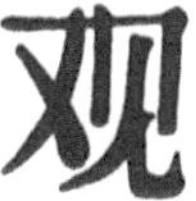

20. K'uan

(Examination)-This Hexagram indicates "examination". The Trigram is a combination of "Sun" and "K'un" and also of wind and earth elements. It is also at total variance with 'Len', because it has two upper lines unbroken and the other four lines are broken ones. This sign is indicative of important and urgent work, or a sort of work upon which sharp eyes of others focused. Hence carefully think of the pros and cons of the matter, before taking up any work. It is also imperative that your decisions should be discreet and serious.

噬嗑

21. Shih Ho

(Beating, Thrashing) — It is also called a hexagon for "Beating". It is a combination of "Li" and "Ch'en," that is there is a combination of fire and electricity elements. In the Trigram there are two unbroken lines on the top, middle and lower sides and also three broken lines. This emblem forewarn about the impending danger (s). For instance excessive indulgence in eating, merry making and luxury could be indicators of danger. You want to possess the desired object there and then but, such a restivity and eagerness can lead you towards misfortune. So, if you desire to attain success, you should have enough of patience.

贲

22. Pi

(Adornable, worth worshipping)—This Hexagram is called as a "Hexagram for adoration." It is a combination of "Ken" and "Li" that is here mountain and fire elements combined. The Trigram is at total variance with "Shih Ho", because there are three broken and three unbroken lines, but positions of earth lines is different. It indicates that every person possesses a peculiar ability in one discipline or the other and that we should recognise and understand his qualities, and we should imbibe his good qualities and translate those into our actions, so that we become adorable. Avoid too much of overspending and also extreme miserlessness, rather adopt a middle path.

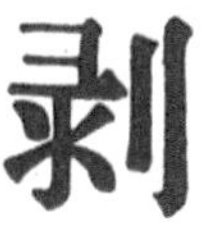

23. PO

(Peeling)— This Hexagram is known as "Peeling Hexagram". It is a combination of"Ken" and "Kun", and earth and mountain elements. First topline looks like a mountain and the other five lines are broken and fall under the first line (mountain) which gives the idea that the mountain is unable to have a solid surface of the earth--- it is indicative of uncertainty which implies that, if one sits on the mountain and relies upon, he will come to grief or taste deceit. It also means that while giving a practical shape to any plan or initiating some new work, do not take any hasty step without analysing the pros and cons, because even a minor modification/deviation in the ongoing work could prove harmful.

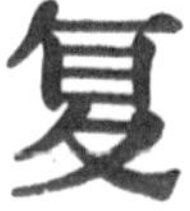

24. Fu

(Return)—This diagram is called a "Return" diagram, and is a combination "Kun" and "Ch'en" and also contains energy (electricity fire). It is totally opposite to 'Po'. In the Trigram only one (lowest) line is unbroken and all other lines are broken. This symbol indicates return or regain of success. It also conveys the message that war is followed by peace and cataclysm by productivity. It is a positive sign also. It is the line when you can improve your damaged works with the help of other people. So do not act in hurry, and let the events take their natural course.

无妄

25. Wu Wang

(Honesty)— This hexagram is known as a 'Hexagram for honesty'. It is made up of 'Chin' and 'Chen' and is also a combination of heaven and energy (electricity). There are two broken and four unbroken lines in this trigram. This symbol motivates and inspires one to follow the course of nature. Do not consider unnecessarily about the works that you can not do. Since you have no control over your fate and natural events, hence whatever you have got, remain satisfied with it and work honestly.

大畜

26. Ta Ch'u

(Have Faith in the Divine and Great Nurturing Power)— This Hexagram is named Hexagon that denotes a divine power capable of nurturing. It is a combination of Ken and Chien and also of mountain and heaven. It is at total variance with Wu Wang. It also has two broken and four unbroken lines but not in the order of lines of Wu Wang. This Trigram denotes that heaven lies beneath the mountain where treasure of (priceless) energy lies hidden. If a person utilises this power for the welfare of others, then he will justify his strength in the form of a nurture.

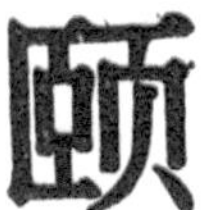

27. Ta Kuo

(Taking Care or Nurturing)___'I' is said to be a hexagon that 'Takes Care or Nurtures." This Trigram is a combination of "Tui and Sun" and marsh and wind element. It consists of two unbroken and four broken lines, that is upper most and lowest line are unbroken while the four broken lines lie in-between the broken lines. Here four broken lines represent Yang energy and these lines are like strong being, but the upper and lower (unbroken) lines are unable to sustain and bear the weight of the beam. This emblem indicates that changes are due to occur in the near future; hence do not waste your energy in future pursuits, rather preserve it to attain favourable results.

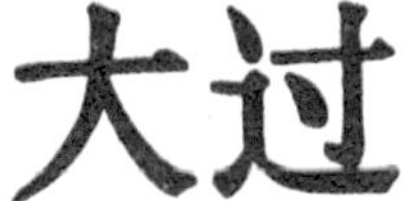

28. I

(Taking care; Nourishing)— This Hexagram, is known as a 'Taking Care Hexagram". The Trigram is a combination of "Ch'en" and "Ken" and of mountain and energy. This Trigram is shaped like a mouth-its upper and lower lines resemble like two lips, and the broken lines denote teeth which lie in between the lips. Mouth wants food, but food can be had when helped by others so such a type of help should be within a reasonable limit. In a way your planning needs to be nurtured and guided properly.

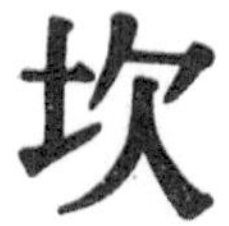

29. K'an

(Watery Depth) — This hexagon is called a "Watery Depth" Hexagram and herein "Ken Trigram and water element have surfaced twice. There are two Yang (unbroken lines) line which give the impression as if a river is flowing without any obstruction. It denotes that you should not be carried away by your hyped ambitions, because you can be carried away and rushed by the strong current of events. Hence focus attention on your objective. The persons, on whom you rely and confide too much, should be relied upon, and face the ordeals with patience.

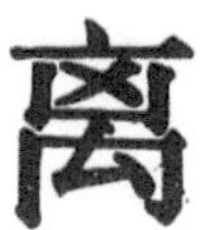

30. Li

(Brilliant Lustre; Shine)— This is called a hexagon of "Bright lustre or Shine". "Li" represents fire element and it has appeared twice in this Trigram. This sign is attributed to light and human civilization, and the light appears in the form of sun light during the day and moonlight at night. Both sunlight and moonlight represent human civilization. This emblem conveys significance of light which implies that you can progress and surge ahead towards your goal, if you coordinate with nature. So, minutely and thoroughly study the situations around you, chalf out a suitable plan, the surge ahead towards your cheerful goal.

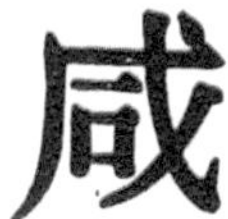

31. Hsien

(Hospitality, Reciprocity)— Hsien is an all embracing hexagon that denotes 'Hospitality and Reciprocity. It is a combined form of "Tui" and "Ken" Trigrams. If fact, it is a combination of marsh and mountain elements. Swamp is found on the mountain which impacts the earth. This emblem is a combination of firm resolve and humility, and both the qualities are needed for productivity. If you can tender advice/to others, you too should be fully prepared to pay heed to the advise of others. Do not surge ahead in a hurry and also do not change your plans. Have the patience, watch the situations all around you, and then proceed. Do not be carried away by reactions, rather welcome the reactions.

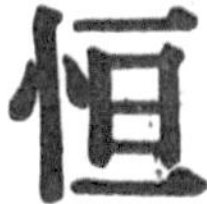

32. Heng

(Constant)— This Hexagram is called 'Constant' which is a combined form of "Chien" and "Sun" Trigrams. In fact, it is a combination of wind element and electricity (energy). It denotes a powerful dual character, that is to say that character changes like the phases of sun and moon, but light does not abjure the sun and moon. Carefully observe the changing demeanour of your friends and foes and also closely study the environment around you, and do not commit the blunder of not understanding the change in persons and situations. Do not also think that you will attain instant success. Patiently wait for and observe the changes in situation, that is, you should not lose patience, rather wait for the advent of favourable solution.

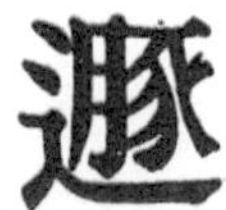

33. Tun

(To Hide)— 'Tun' is known as a "Hiding" Hexagram which is a union of "Chien" and "Ken" Trigrams. This, in fact, denotes a union of mountain and heaven. The Trigram has four unbroken lines on the upper side and two broken lines down side. Lower broken lines are the 'Yin' lines and the four unbroken lines are 'Yang" lines. It also implies that it is the time to contemplate and think and not to act: If you are planning to give a practical shape to any plan, then wait and do not proceed in a hurry, rather carefully assess the hidden dangers.

大壮

34. Ta Chuang

(Great Strength)— Ta Chung Hexagram is known as a "Trigram of great success". The Trigram is a combination of "Chien" and "Chien" which actually denotes lesson of electricity (power, energy) and heaven. This Trigram is totally opposite to 'Tun' Trigram, because there are two broken lines on the upper sides and four unbroken lines on the lower side- the broken lines stand for Yen and unbroken lines for 'Yang" lines. Power of electricity ably benefits and works for the intrinsic power of heaven. So, it is an appropriate line that favours you, even if fear, doubts or hallucinations openly surface but such factors must not discourage or dissuade you. Take full advantage of great power, but do not be overtaken, by other confidence.

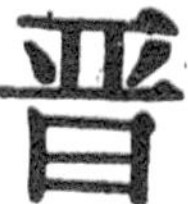

35. Chin

(Advance)— This Hexagram has been named as an "Advance Hexagram" which is a unified form of " Li" and "Kien" Trigrams which, in fact, denotes as coordinated combination of fire and earth elements. This trigram consists of two unbroken lines and four broken lines. This is the most appropriate time when you can give a practical shape to your plans. As you expectations and ambitions are quite high you may find it a bit difficult task to perform. This sign also indicates progress and auspicious sign. But you must share your fortune (which has come to you well in advance) with your well wishers and friends. Hence also create such a favourable environment where feelings and ideas of others could also be accommodated.

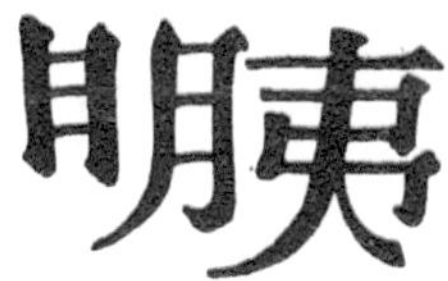

36. MingI

(Opaqueness, Dimmed Brightness)— This Hexagram is a combination of"Ken" and "Li" Trigrams which, in fact, is a combination of earth and fire elements. It is a converse Trigram of "Chein". It has also four broken and two unbroken lines but are placed in different positions. In this emblem, light of fire is wrapped with darkness due to shadow of the earth. Hence, the lines is full of hallucinations for Yen. You are incapable of taking final decision on any matter. Yen should take your own time in deciding how to implement your plans, and should not be carried away by emotive feelings. If you are overpowered by another person's pressure, then listen to the voice of your conscience and decided according to your own direction and thinking.

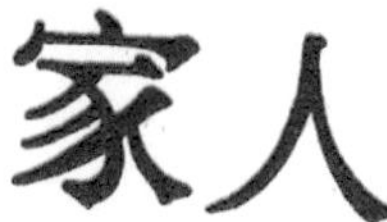

37. Chia Jen

(The Family) — This is known as a 'Family' Hexagram. The diagram is formed by union of "Sun" and "Li" diagrams, and is a combination of wind and fire elements. We all are influenced by the women folk. There is no coordination between the neighbours and environs around you, and such a coordination is utmost necessity. You should not be only concerned with your own self, rather you should also consider those persons who live with you and also stand by you. Keep a watch on your home and environs around you.

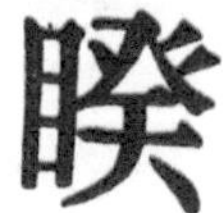

38. K'uei

(Opposition)— This is a Hexagram of opposition which is a unified form of "Li" and "Tui" diagram, and is also a combined form of fire and swamp, It is totally opposite to "Chia Jen" diagram, as fire and swamp are totally opposed to each other-- flames of fire rise upwards, whereas swamp flows downwards. Hence natural friendship and partnership between the two elements can not go hand-in-hand. Since this is a period of uncertainty, you should exert control over yourself and fix your attention on your target and the proceed towards completion of your plans.

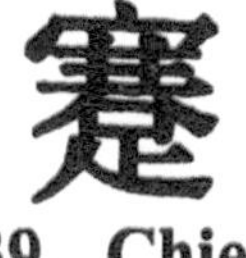

39. Chien

(Difficulty)— This Hexagram is a unified form of 'K'an' and "Ken" diagram and is also a combination of mountain and water elements. It consists of two unbroken and four broken lines. You should study the environs around you, before you waste your strength and squander your money. You should focus your attention on anticipated and imminent difficulties and problems, but do not prolong the course of contemplation, nor give a long rope to your plans otherwise you will lose your courage and thrust. So, seek the advice of other persons and it is possible their advice may prove productive and useful to enable you to wriggle out of the impasse.

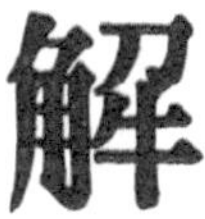

40. H Sieh

(Release, Freedom)— This Hexagram is made up by the combination of "Ch'ien" and "Kan" diagrams, and combination of water and electricity elements. Its position is reverse of "Chien" diagram, thought there are two unbroken and four broken lines in each of Chien and H Sieh diagrams, yet they are posted in variant positions. This emblem helps a person to extricate himself from problems. The lines in this diagram convey the impression as if open sky has been purified consequent upon thundering of clouds, storm and rainfall. It suggest that time is right for taking a decision. However, there is no harm in taking others opinions.

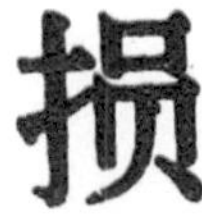

41. Sun

(Better Lines)— 'Sun' Hexagram is a unified form of "Ken" and "Tui" diagrams. It is also a combined form of swamp and mountains elements. It consists of three broken and three unbroken lines. This emblem indicates that your fortune is on the verge of change for the better. Although you have already spent away plenty of time and money, but now the time has come when your outstandings will get cleared. You will be fully satisfied by complete recovery of your outstanding dues and also that the money, spent in new works or plan, is completely secured and protected.

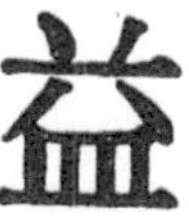

42. I

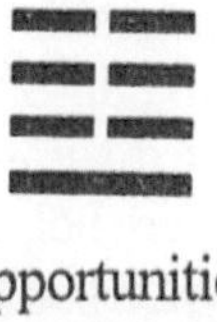

"I" diagram is composed by combination of "Sun" and "Chen". Its elements are electricity and wind. This diagram is totally the opposite of "Sun" diagram. This sign indicates cooperation and change to better time. There is a possibility of change of place. All the hurdles and bottlenecks in the way of progress will be dispelled and you will have suitable opportunities for making progress. You do not have to explain your waves and plans to any other person, since all the obstacles have been removed, possibilities of progress are in plenty and you can surge ahead towards your targeted path.

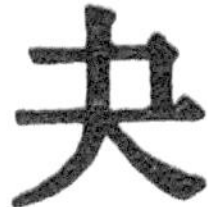

43. Kuai

(New gains, Outcome)— Kuai Hexagram is made up by combining "Tui" and "Chi'en" diagrams. It is also a meeting place of swamp and heaven. Here first line is broken and other five lines are unbroken. This emblem indicates that the phase of heavy rains and typhoon has already blown over and the new way has been paved-this development indicates possibility of new gain or object. Hence, it is most suitable to proceed on the path of progress and use the rest of the life in attempts to take opportunities for gains.

姤

44. Kou

(Meeting, Joining)—Kou Hexagram is a combination of "Chien" and "Sun" diagram and also of heaven and wind elements. It is totally reversed of "Kuo" diagram. Herein there is one broken lines at the bottom and five unbroken lines are sighted upon this line, whereas, in "Kaui" there is one broken line and five unbroken lines lies thereunder. It indicates that new and favourable opportunities have joined hands for the better and you will be able to adopt yourself according to the situation. But you must ensure that change is beneficial and that you have analysed all the merits and demerits of the changer.

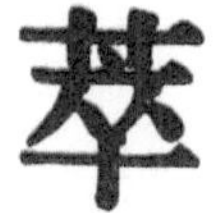

45. T' Sui

(To Collect, Accumulate)— This Hexagram is a combined form of "Tui" and "Kun" diagrams. It is also the diagram where marsh and earth elements combine each other. This diagram indicates that full and complete attention must be paid to minutely and completely understand the environs around you. Try to convert such an atmosphere in your favour. Take your own time and do not jump into conclusions in haste.

升

46. Sheng

(To Progress, Proceed)— Sheng is an unified form of "Kun" and "Sun" and earth and wind elements also meet here. This emblem is reverse of 'T' Sui' diagram where also, there are two broken and four unbroken lines, but their descending orders varies. This emblem resembles a seed which is ripe and awaiting to blossom and emerge in the form of tree. The seed grows into a full-fledged tree, the form has to wait patiently till it finally grows into a tree-this indication points out that situation is favourable and chances for achieving progress will also come up. Since an opportunity advantage from the opportunity.

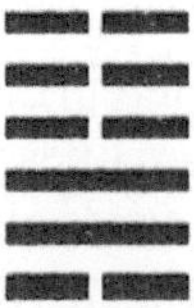

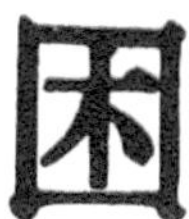

47. K'un

(Surrounded by Problems)— In this Hexagram there is a combination of "Tui" and "Ken" diagrams where swamp and water elements also combine. These combinations imply imprisonment, from which it is extremely difficult for a person to free himself. Though there is a faint hope of freeing one self, yet the incumbent should thoroughly study the situation existing all around. This emblem warns a person to avoid wasteful spending, keep control over precipitatory factors and remain guarded against future (events), and analyse carefully the existing situations and then surge ahead.

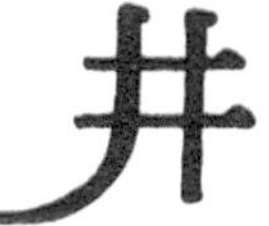

48. Ching

(Deep waters or The well) — This Hexagram is combination of "Kan" and "Sun" and wind water elements also combine herein. This diagram is at a total variance with "K'un" diagram. This emblem indicates to our relationship with nature. If we fail to fully understand the natural circumstances, we will be deprived of the benefits of nature's powerful resources. Hence, feel and realize the favourability or otherwise of the environs around you, by studying the mountains, plants, their shape and forms and colours.

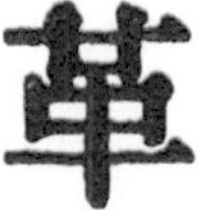

49. Ko

(Change)— "Ko" Hexagram is a unified entity of "Tu" or "Li" and also of fire and swamp elements. This sign/denotes balance between failure and success. It tells, wait for the right opportunity to knock at your door. Before you initiate any activity or work, you must ensure that the time, place and circumstances are fully favourable and beneficial, otherwise you may come with grief.

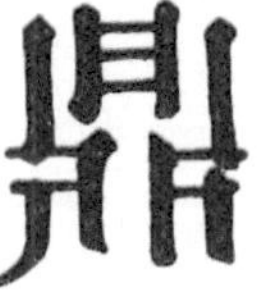

50. Tiug

(Cooking Pot)___ This Hexagram is a unified combination of "Tui" and "Li" diagrams and also of fire and water elements, where there are two broken and four broken lines, but position of all the lines varies in both the diagrams. This emblem is indicative of the food that has been fully cooked on fire, and good utensils are required to cook tasty food. Similarly, one's own experience and help of good friends is needed to initiate any new project in an effective and impressive way.

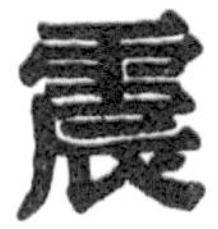

51. Chen

(Shock or Jerk)—As Chen Hexagram is composed of "Chen" electric element has emerged twice herein. There is a hearsay in China that electricity was the causative factor in the Chinese emperor's birth. They wanted to render earth and heaven from their respective places. So, this sign denotes firm determination, pledge and power at their zenith, So, do not be scared of sudden shocks (reverses), not even get nervous due to any event that occurs suddenly. So, if you rely upon and use your intellect, such unexpected and sudden events and shocks can prove beneficial and productive.

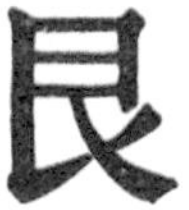

52. Ken

Resting—This Hexagram is made up of "Ken" diagram where "Ken" has appeared twice which indicates mountain element. This Trigram is reverse to "Chen". This mountain is reflective with power and peace, where animals and plants are taking rest. So, this sign indicates one should relax and take rest, by giving proper rest to your own decisions.

漸

53. Chien

(Slow Progress)— This Hexagram is formed by combination of "Sun" and "Ken" Trigram and here wind and mountain elements are also unified. There are two unbroken lines at the top and two broken lines at the lower end, and there also exists a broken and unbroken line each in between the said upper and lower lines. So that there exists three broken and three unbroken lines. This sign suggest do not undervalue the gains you have acquired through your own experiences. So, patience and wisdom are of utmost necessity, otherwise you will prove yourself wrong. It is better to seek advice of others and then steadily proceed on the path of progress.

归妹

54. Kuei Mei

(Marriage, Happiness)—Kue Mei Hexagram is a unified form of "Chen" and "Tui" Trigrams which also indicates combination of electric and swamp elements. Kuei Mei is totally an opposite of "Chien". In this Trigram, there are two broken lines at the top, then an unbroken line, then a broken line and lastly two unbroken lines-that is, there are three broken and three unbroken lines. This sign points out to coordination between positive and negative family relations. Hence all feuds and egoism should be removed as quickly as possible. Try also to rectify mistakes, as delay and apathy will add to further problems. Hence, use your description as to in which situation you have to speak the bitter truth or where to deny.

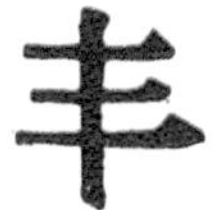

55. Feng

(Prosperity, Progress)— This Hexagram is composed of union of "Che'n" and "Li" Trigrams, and it is also a combination of electric and fire elements. This sign indicates healthy progress and strength. It is the light that brightens the earth and light of electricity brightens the sky. Hence, you need to be afraid at all, as the time has changed for the better and all hurdles on the ways to your progress have got removed. The decisions which are best suited now may not prove fruitful the next day, so, do not worry unnecessarily on this score, because change is the law of nature. Do whatever you consider as the best option for achieving progress and objective of your own.

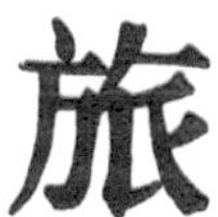

56. Lu

(Travelling)— This Hexagram is a unified and combined form of "Li" and "Ken" Trigrams. This Trigram also points out to fire and mountain elements. Travelling and change in travelling are the main indications of this Trigram. It generally happens in life that you are required to visit an unknown place, and it does take long to acquaint oneself with the new place. Remain cautious and alert. Do not expose yourself as long as you do not acquaint yourself fully to the other persons in that area.

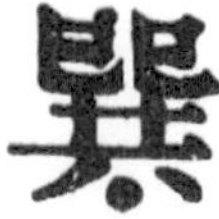

57. Sun

(Gentility, Civility)— This Hexagon is indicative of wind element and "Sun" appears herein twice. It is not possible to avoid the impact and flow of wind so, it is not wise to stand against the flow of wind. Fierce storm uproots and decinates even the big trees, but humble grass get neither disturbed nor uprooted due to its low lying profile which, in fact, denotes its humility. In adverse circumstances you should rely upon humility and gentility. If you do so, you can achieve your targeted objective. So, never swim against the tide, adopt a low profile by remaining gentle and humble, instead of taking to the path of confrontation.

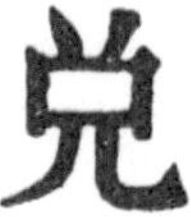

58. Tui

(Happiness)— This Hexagon is reverse of the "Tui" Trigram, "Tui" represents swamp. In this Trigram "Tui" has surfaced twice and the sign represents optimism. If we accept the ground realities of existing circumstances, which are staring us in the face, then every situation will prove favourable. Hence accept the present situation with a receptive and cheerful mind. This is the secret of your success, provided you move patiently and be satisfied with present lot. You should try to recognise and enhance your positive faculties.

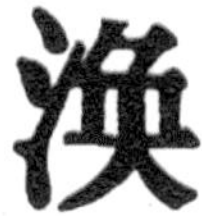

59. Huan

(Scatter, Separate)---"Huan" Hexagram is a conglomerated form of "Sun" and "Ken" Trigrams and its elements are wind and air. As wind disturbs a lake's clean water, by creating tumult, so do sudden emblem denotes separation and it also scatters. Hence, you should patiently wait for congenial normalcy of nature, as sudden changes will open the gateway to new possibilities. So, apply your intellect at a faster pace.

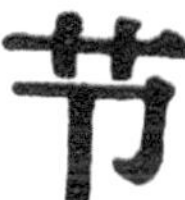

60. Chieh

(Limitation)—"Chief" Hexagram is a unified form of "Tui" and "Ken"diagrams, and it represents swap and water elements also. It is totally reverse of "Huan" Trigram. Abnormal flow of water can cause both famine and floods, hence water flow should be kept under normal control, that is, water should not be the cause of famine or floods. This sign indicates that in our practical life also we should maintain suitable balance between extreme zeal. So, do not become a stone-hearted human nor be so humble that you resort to cowardice. This sign also induces self-restraints and, then, take to the middle path.

中孚

61. Chung Fu

(Inner Confidence)—It is a unified combination form of "Sung" and "Tui" Trigrams which also represents swamp and air elements. This sign emblem indicates that it is nature that provides success and access to auspicious things, hence do not be restive and desponded, rather control your feelings and requirements. You should not also forget and ignore your friends. Keep your internal confidence on high pedestal, and whatever work you do, with complete confidence and zeal.

小过

62. Hsio Kuo

(Minor Problem)—This Hexagram is a conglomeration of "Chien" and "Ken" Trigrams, and also a combination of electric and mountain element. This sign has four broken (Yen) lines and two unbroken lines which indicate that there are multiple illusory fallacies which give rise to many problems. So, do not think that whatever you are doing is correct and in order. But you must know life and its problems can provide you experience at every step. Hence, whatever step you take, move slowly as at every step you can learn something.

既济

63. Chi Chi

(Finalised, Completed)—This Hexagram is a combination of "Ken" and "Li" Trigrams and it also denotes combination of water and fire elements, we can work effectively, by utilising faculties of these elements. You should also know that art of taking work out of the two divergent elements. If you complete a job, never think is an end of your working. It is not good to cherish a feeling that you have finished your work because everchanging circumstances and challenges lie ahead. So, do not take a pause, rather keep on working.

未济

64. Wei Chi

(Not Yet done)—This Hexagon is a combination of "Kun" and "Li" Trigrams and also of fire and water elements. It is also at total variance with "Chi Chi" Trigram. Water and fire elements are natural enemies to each other. Struggle is staring you in your face; hence you should remain alert and cautious, and do not unpose your own plans on any other person, nor even your plans and working. The only mantra for success lies in mutual cooperation and patience. If your plans are proper and you have patience, you shall emerge victorious in your objective.

❑❑❑

PART–3
Advance Feng Shui

9
Five Elements in Feng Shui

Chinese Vaastu Shastra believes in five elements, like Indian. The Chinese believe that all living species, including humans, mountain, vegetation or for that matter whatever we observe in this universe are made of these five elements. Once a person fully understands the secrets and diverse factors inherent in five elements. He, can fully know what Chinese scholars expounded in the practice of Feng Shui. Because emergence and end of the universe is guided by these elements which also impact our routined life.

Five elements are mentioned hereunder-

English	Chinese	Signs	Meaning of the signs
WOOD	Mu	I-L	Vertical line or L Shape
FIRE	Huo	Λ Δ	Triangle
WATER	Shui	≈	Waves
METAL	Chin	(O	Semi-Circle or Circle.
EARTH	Tu	□ ⊓	Quadrangle

Analysis of Elements

1. WOOD ELEMENT

All the trees, vegetable, leaves, paper and furniture represent the wood element. All those objects which are green or related to green colour, whether it be a green coloured wall or any other thing, get observed into wood element. Direction of this element is east and its season is spring season.

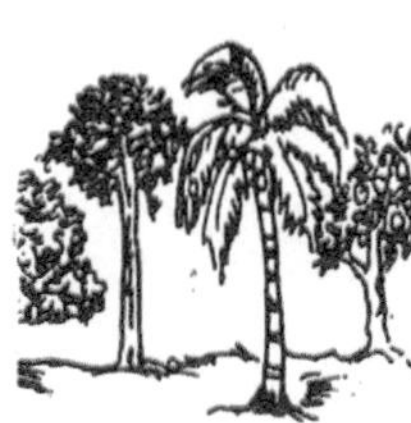

Direction for red or white coloured wood is south-east ('Agni kone'). According to numerology '3' and '4' numbers represent wood element, according to Chinese astrology "Tiger" and "Hare" animals represent wood element. A vertical or L-shaped figure denoted wood element.

2. FIRE ELEMENT

Colour of fire is red, orange or saffron. It enhances 'Yang' energy. Its season is summer and direction is south. Sharp light represents fire element. According to Chinese astrology "Snake" and "Horse" signs are representatives of fire element. A triangular shape form is indicative of the fire element.

3. WATER ELEMENT

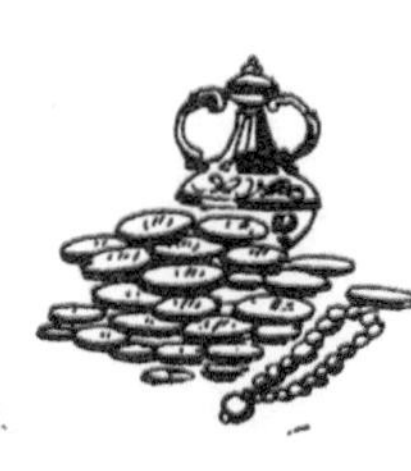

Colour of water element is blue, sky blue or black. It occupies the eastern direction and its season is winter. Water enhances 'Yin' energy. According to numerology number "1" represents water element. All the sources of water, like oceans, rivers water ponds, water falls, wells, fountains, fish aquariums etc. submerge into water element. According to Chinese astrology zodiac signs of "Mouse" and "Pig" represent the water element.

4. METAL ELEMENT

All types of metal make the element. Its colour is yellow, golden, white, copper like, and black like iron, including all the colours of alloys. It occupies western direction and its season is rainy season. Direction of east is the direction for small metals. According to numerology numbers "6" and "7" represents metal element. According to Chinese astrology the metal element is represented through bells, wind-chimneys, coins and ornaments.

5. EARTH ELEMENT

Colour of earth resembles grey or brown colour or earthen colour. Every part of land is the representative of earth element. Third month of every season is influenced

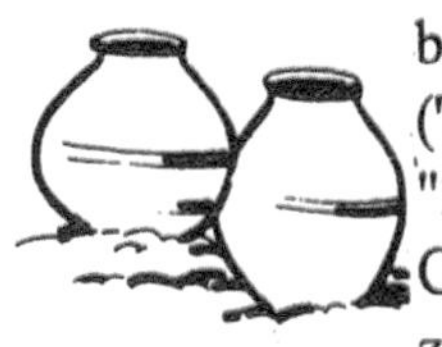

by earth element. This element occupies. South-West ('Naireitya') direction. According to numerology numbers "2", "5" and "8" represent earth element. According to Chinese astrology "Buffalo", "Goat", "Dragon" and "Dog" zodiac signs represent earth element.

Mutual affinity and relationship amongst the elements

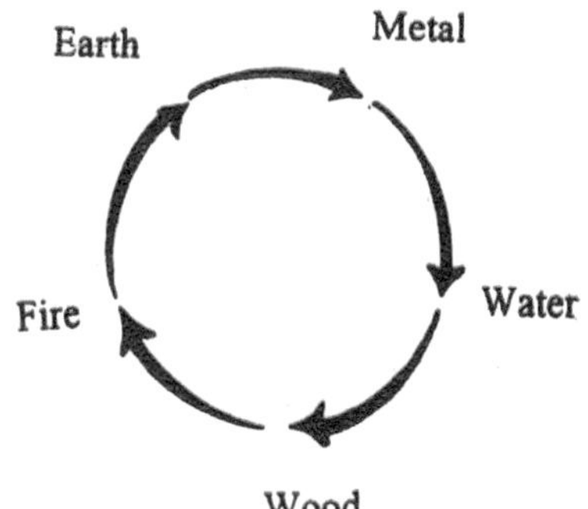

1. When Fire+Earth elements combine, fire-balls get converted into earth elements by the help of volcano(s).
2. When Earth+Metal elements combine, all the metals lying in the womb of earth, generate metal mines and represent metals.
3. If Metal+Water combine, metal melts and, thus, gets liquified, and it is the water element that imparts solidity to metals.
4. Combination of Water+Wood results in the growth of plants, trees and vegetables which yield woods, as wood can not be had unless the plants are nurture and saturated by water.
5. Wood generates fire, because when wood is burnt we get fire.

How an element destroys or harms another element

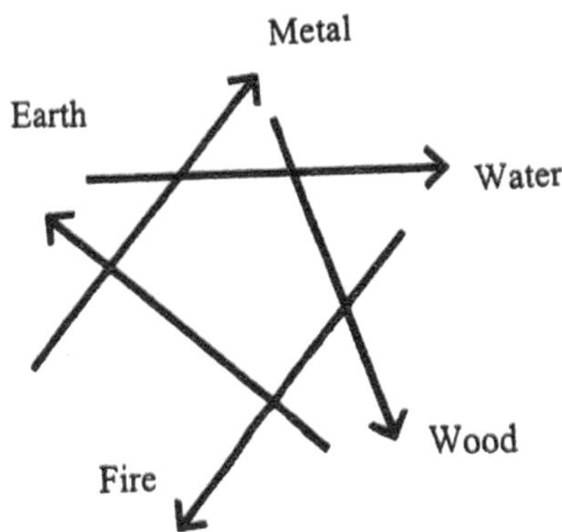

- Water is polluted by earth
- Water mollifies/extinguishes fire
- Fire melts metal
- Metal cuts wood
- Wood harms the earth

Each element is dependent upon its preceding element. Similarly, every element is also controlled by the element, form which it has generated. A controlling element is that which destroys or deciumates a harming element or generates that element. Which destroys the energy of the element that causes harm.

For instance, there is a room which has green coloured walls, its furniture is also of green colour and the carpet, spread on the surface, is also green. Too much use and adherence to the green colour definitely casts its influence on the native. Such a person will live in the world of imagination, because he will be far away from the realities of life. In order to offset or dilute damaging impact of excessive green colour, white or red coloured furniture or carpet should be used. White colour represents metal element which, in fact, destroys wood elements. Hence it will neutralise and balance excessive impact of wood element. Similarly, red colour is indicative of fire element, and red colour will establish equilibrium and harmony, for the simple reason that it is the wood that generates fire, as fire ignites itself to produce fire.

Controlled Elements

Harmful elements	Controlled elements	
	Constructive	Destructive
1. Water	Wood	Earth
2. Wood	Fire	Metal
3. Fire	Earth	Water
4. Earth	Metal	Wood
5. Metal	Water	Fire

Any object we observe in this universe decidedly represent one element or the other. Destructive an harmful effects can be brought under control by using a controlling element. Following is the list of signifying objects of earth element.

Element	Signifying objects
Wood	Green colour, green plants flower pot, wood or (wooden) furniture
Fire	Red colour, light, a cloth of red colour
Earth	Picture of yellow colour, yellow cloth in plants in an earthen pot.
Metal	Articles processed from white colour or white metal.
Water	Black colour, fountain or aquarium.

Characteristics of Persons (according to five elements)

1. Characteristic of natives with Earth element

Persons, whose representative element is the earth, are faithful to their masters, have an idealistic character but are highly ambitious. These persons have dual character. They wish and desire that other persons should pay importance to them, and they desire loving treatment. They should stay away from moisture marshy lands, cold and watery places.

2. Characteristic of natures having Fire element

Persons of fire element have magnetic and attractive personality, remain happy and excited. They wish to remain bound in love of relatives, as they despise seclusion. They are hyper sensitiveand quick messengers. They should avoid hyper emotivity and places where there is too much heat.

3. Characteristics of nature having Metal element

They are excellent calculators. They wish to land an orderly and principled life. They also like hygienic atmosphere. Quality is the creed of their life, they should avoid dry places.

4. Characteristic of nature having Water element

Such persons, whose element is water, are imaginative, philosophers and thinkers. They are clever, scholarly and believe in freelancing. They take up multiple professions. They believe in conferring secrets to themselves only. They should avoid water logged places.

5. Characteristic of nature having Wood element

They are high class artists and perform diligently committed to their profession. They wish to remain busy and believe in the sort of life which is labour oriented. They indulge is wasteful spending. They should avoid such places where strong winds blow.

Variable factors between five elements of indian Vaastu Shastra and Chinese Feng Shui

In Feng Shui five elements, such as, 1. Wood, 2. Fire, 3. Water, 4. Metal, 5. Earth elements are considered as causative factors in the certain of the universe whereas in Indian Vaastu Shastra1. Earth, 2.Water, 3. Fire, 4. Wind and 5. Akash (Vaccum or Space) are considered as the contributory factors that create universe. Indian view point is more scientific, because infusion of life is not possible without wind in all the movable and immovable species, so it is the case with existence of space.

In Feng Shui, wood, metal and earth are considered as separate elements, whereas wood and metal elements generate from earth and then, ultimately submerge into earth itself. All the plants, trees stones dust, gold, silver, mountains, brass, jewels and diamonds, coal, ash are simply modified forms of earth in a way these are the bi-product of earth. Hence all the said objects have no independent existence of earth and this assertion is fully backed by scientific reality. It is only the Indian scholars who gave to the universe the concept of 'Panch bhootas (five elements), and in particular 'Space' and 'Wind'. Hence, Indian Vaastu science is, by far, the last and highest philosophy which is leased in, formed resourcing and philosophy.

❑❑❑

10
Lo-Shu—The Magical Square

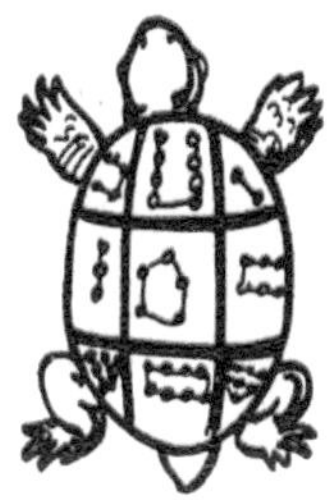

Concept of 'Lo-Shu' as a magical square was conceived about 4000 B.C. when a large-sized tortoise emerged out of 'Lo' river. China's principle national river. The hard shell (cover) of the tortoise was seen compartmentalized into eight squares, and some protruding dots were also observed emerging on each of the squares.

It was indeed a magical light that the total number of figures in three squares or aggregated to 15, even if counted from any side, horizontally or vertically. At the time counting of numerical figures had just began and emergence of 'Lo-Shu' was a magical appearance which became an inseparable part of Chinese religion 'Taoism'. The subject tortoise is considered as one of the four divine animals as it is considered lord of eastern direction.

Use of Lo-Shu in Feng Shui

4 Early South East	9 Fire Summer	2 Late Summer
3 Wood Spring East	5 Earth	7 Metal Autumn West
8 Late North East	1 Water Winter North	6 Early Winter North West

Use of Lo-Shui is scintillating. Magical squares became more rampant in Feng Shui and it was considered a divine power. If you closely look at the above square, you can easily find earth element in grey colour No. 5, No. 9 is red colour above it and water element at No. 1 in blue colour below it, wood element is found in green colour at 3, and metal element in yellow colour at No. 7.

So, such a meaningful conclusion of imaging 5 elements in the square is aligned to the Chinese base principles of Feng Shui.

4 Early Summer South East	9 Fire Summer South	2 Late Summer South West
3 Wood Spring East	5 Earth	7 Metal Autumn West
8 Late Winter North East	1 Water Winter North	6 Early Winter North West

Such an imaginative concept assumed more significant and explicit portents when the Feng Shui experts alleged directions and seasons also to 'Lou-Shu' magical square. The uniqueness of this square lies in its faculty to point out Southern direction on the upper side, whereas in compass North is always indicated on the top side.

In Chinese Feng Shui, hanging of 'Lo-Shu' emblem on shops and business houses is considered very auspicious. There is nothing new in magic of 'Lo-Shu' but it is simply a rebash of much famous 'Panariya Yantra' which is awakened and sanctified with chant of relevant mantras. Similarly, in India 'Beesa Yantra' in another magical emulate and the total in all the squares will come to 20, whether calculated from upside, down side or diagonally.

Feng-Shui of a House according to Lo-Shui

4 PROPERTY FORTUNE SE	9 RESPECT S	2 MARRIAGE SW
3 AFFECTION OF MOTHER & ELDERS E	5 HEALTH	7 CHILDREN W
8 EDUCATION NE	1 CAREER N	6 FRIENDLY AIDE NW

Plan of Eastern Door according to Lo-Shui or Ba-gua Divine or Godly Benevolence

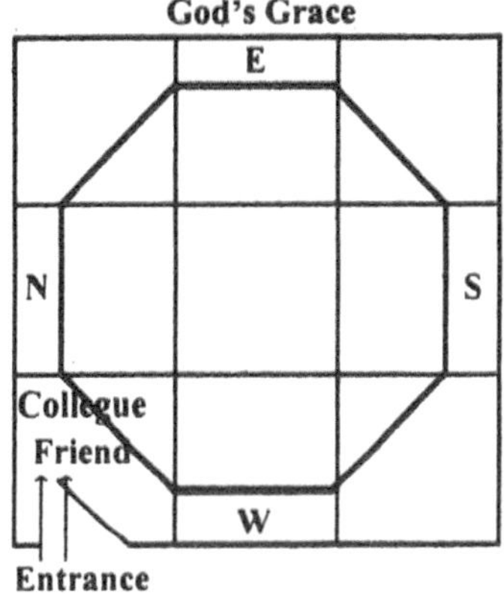

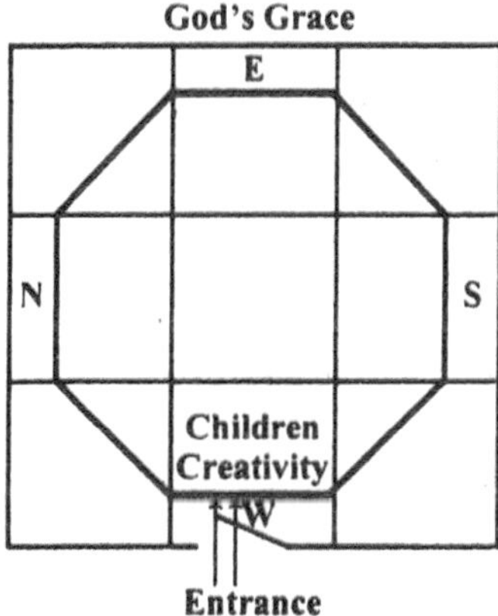

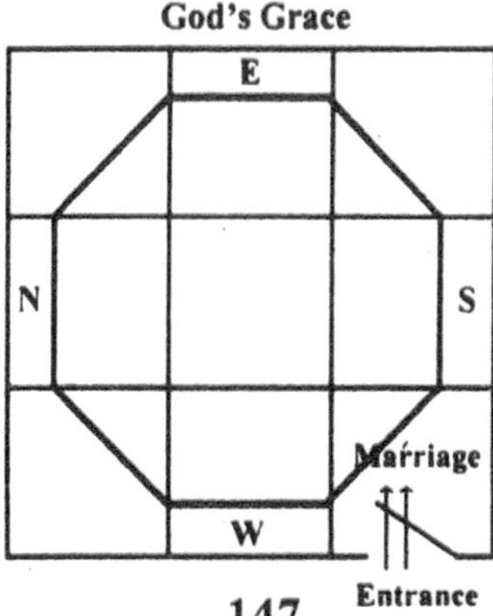

Plan of Southern Gate according to Lo-Shui or Ba-gua Fame & Reputation

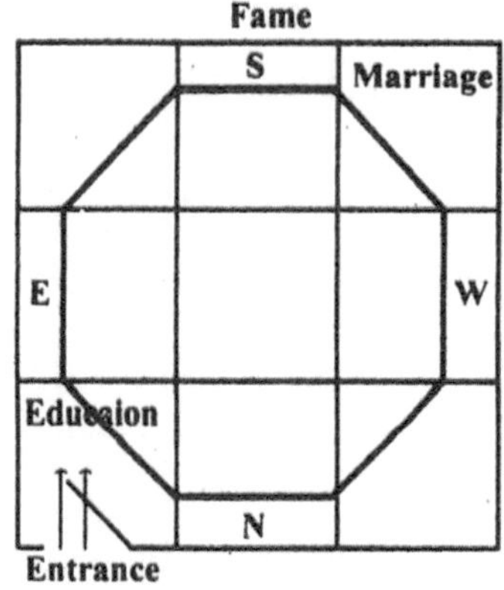

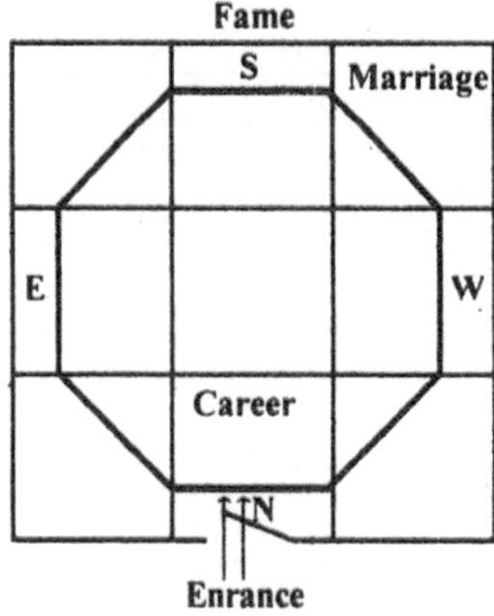

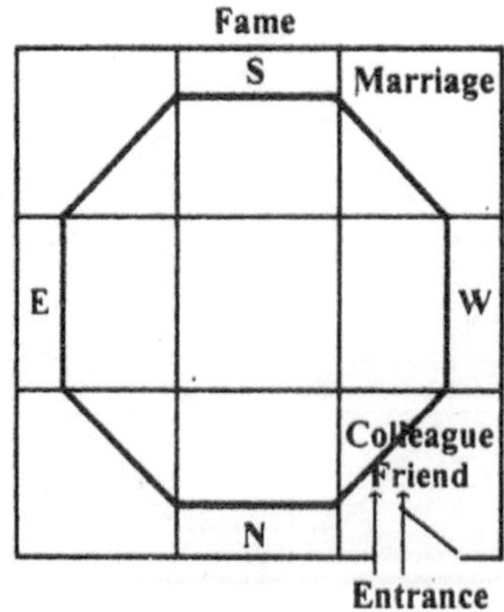

Plan of Northern Gate according to Feng-Shui or Ba-gua

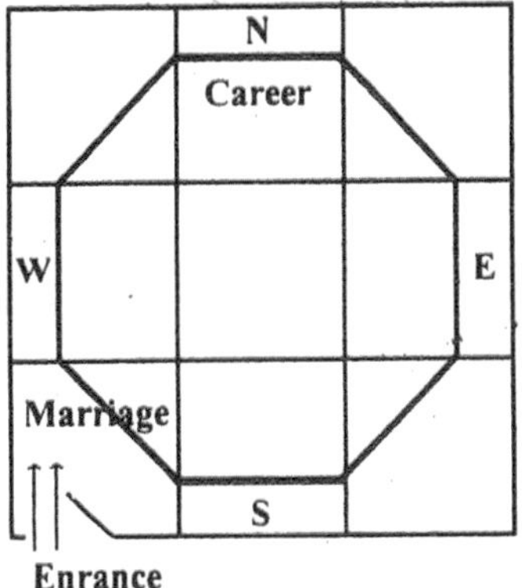

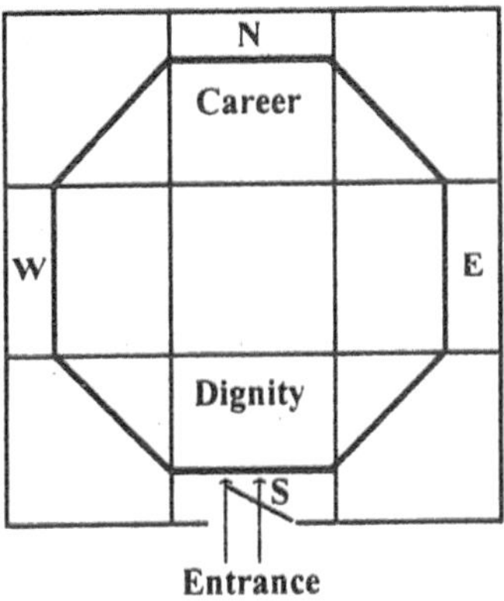

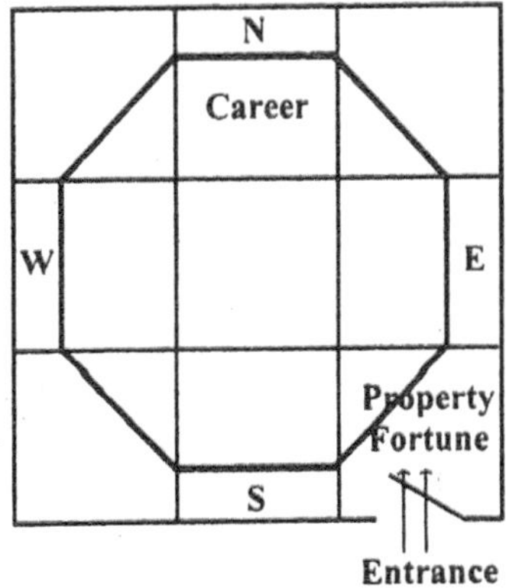

Plan of Western Gate according to Lo -Shu and Ba-gua Progeny

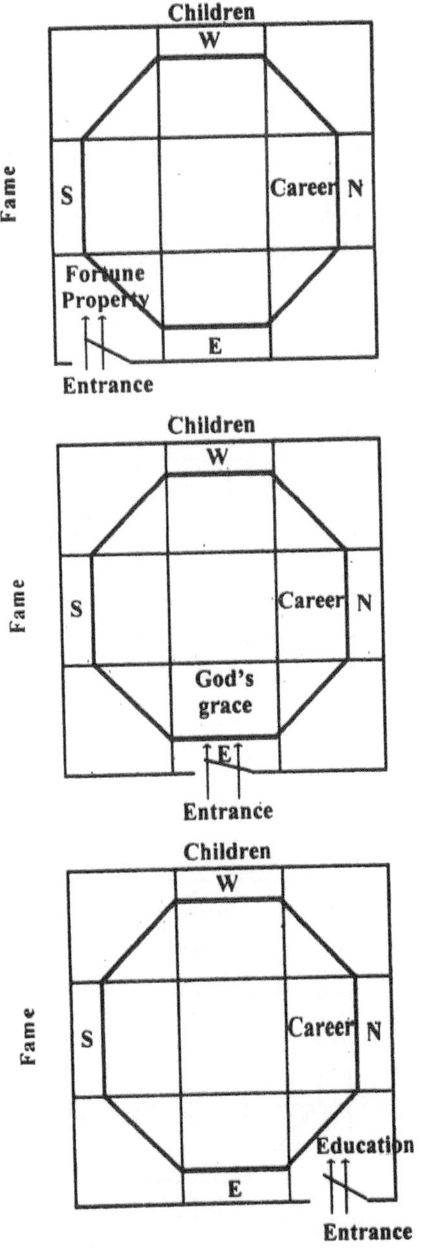

11
Star Feng Shui

Position of zodiac sign and astro-signs (nakhshatras) existing at the time of the birth is examined to learn the defects related to direction in Feng Shui. Directional evils or faults can be rectified by simple corrective devices. Panaruja Yantra is the basis of Feng Shui where the basis is five elements and eight directions.

Eight Direction

1. East 2. West 3. North 4. South 5. North-East (Ishanya) 6. South East (Agnikona) 7. South-West (Nairitya) and 8. North-West (Vaayavya)

Five Elements

1. Water element : Its representative digit is = 1
2. Earth element : Its representative digit is = 2,5,8
3. Wood element : Its representative digit is = 3,4
4. Metal element : Its representative digit is = 6,7
5. Fire element : Its representative digit is = 9.

4 SE	9 S	2 SW
E 3	Centre 5	W 7
NE 8	N 1	NW 6

Mention date of birth of a person within this Panariya yantra in place of and at the exact designated place, and then see for yourself the magical outcome. For instance, if a person is born on 4-9-1994, the figures should be inserted in the yantra as detailed here under-

SE 44	S 999	SW
E	Centre	W
NE	1 N	NW

Resultant outcome

(A) Numbers 2,5 and 8, which represent earth element, are missing which implies that the persons's relations and family are weak and he is a weak person. His relatives will not help him in his progress. Overconfidence will prove counter productive and he will be ditched. He will never be rewarded in proportion to his ability and efforts.

Remedy

1. Keep a lamp of yellow coloured light in the centre of the house.
2. Paste pictures of mountains in the south-west direction.
3. Dangle two pictures of mountains in the bed-room also.

The aforesaid remedial steps will improve weak status or condition of earth element.

(B) Numbers '6' and '7' represent metal element which denotes the person will always feel the absence of real and sincere friends and relatives, and he has to work hard in order to enjoy fruits of his luck.

Remedy

Number of good friends will enhance if a bracelet or bangle of yellow metal is worn on the right hand. If ladies wear golden bangles, number of their friends will also enhance.

(C) In this chart digits 2,7 and 6 lines are completely missing, such persons will always hesitate to seek help from other persons.

Remedial methods:

Deficiency of Water element

1. Keep a utensil filled with water in the east or north-east direction.
2. Open a water-hut, donate water, serve water to the thirsty.

Deficiency of Earth element

1. Keep heavy articles in the south-west direction.
2. Fortify and strengthen wall in the south-west corner.
3. Dangle/pictures of mountains in the south-west corner.
4. Construct your bed-room in the south-west direction.

Deficiency of Wood element

1. Keep the north-east corner of your house neat and clean.
2. Dangle a musical chime at the gate.
3. Place small flower pots, having small plants, in the north-east of eastern direction.

Deficiency of Metal element

Wear a golden bangle (of gold) ora bracelet in the right hand.

Deficiency of Fire element

1. Keep your hearth in the south-east corner.
2. Keep a red lamp in the south-east corner.
3. Keep a flower pot, having red flowers in your drawing room.

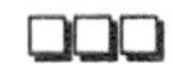

12
Individual auspicious direction and 'Kua' Number

Before we discuss benefits, that are likely to occur, in accordance with Chinese Vaastu Shastra (Feng Shui), it is necessary to know your Kua number's . By 'Kua number' we mean you should know well which of eight directions is the most suited for you, which type of piece building or plot is lucky, where to sit, sleep and reside and which corner of the house is favourable and beneficial, and which are ominous places where you can sit so as to avoid inauspicious results—all such information and guidance is yielded from your Kua number which you will obtain from the following chart. Hereunder, I am explaining the secret formulae, which are rank, for the benefit to discerning readers. It will help you to find out the most suitable spot in the house or piece of land where you can sit, by selecting the most beneficial and useful spot. So that you can make the best use of the auspicious spot.

Secret of Kua number

Add the pair of two digits to the later part of your year of birth, and continue to do so until the remainder comes to "1". The male inmates should deduct the resultant from '10' number, and the restultant final figure will be your Kua number.

The ladies should add '5' to this unit and the resultant final figure will be their Kua number. An example given at the end of this chart, will fully expalin the aforesaid formula.

Illustration

Suppose you were born in 1949, hence the later number is 49= 13 and 1+3 = 4, so, the finaly yield is digit 4.

If you are a male, deduct 4 from 10 the remainder will come to '6' (10-4 = 6). If you are a female, add 4 to 5, and, thus your Kua number will be '9' (4+5), and that of the male will be '6'.

If you study the chart below in the light of the final numbers, you will obtain following results regarding Kua number '6' for a male.

Your KUA Number	1	2	3	4	5 *	6	7	8	9
Lucky Direcion									
Your Shena chi **Success Direction**	SE	NE	S	N	NE* SW	W	NW	SW	E
Your tien yi **Healthy Direction**	E	W	N	S	W	NE	SW	NW	SE
Your Dien yen **Marriage Direction**	S	NW	SE	E	NW W	SW	NE	W	N
Your fu wei **Self ProgressDirection**	N	SW	E	SE	SW NE	NW	W	NE	S
Unlucky Direcion									
Your ho hai **Unlucky Direction**	W	E	SW	NW	E S	SE	N	S	NE
Your we kwei **Ghost Direction**	NE	SE	NW	SW	SE N	E	S	N	W
Your fui sha **Fatal Direction**	NW	S	NE	W	S E	N	SE	E	SW
Your chueh ming **Direction of Loss**	SW	N	W	NE	N SE	S	E	SE	NW

According to Kua number '6', western direction forebodes success, north-east direction imparts fine health, south-west enhances love and affection and north-west is the best direction for personal progress.

In the case of females, No '9' indicates —east imparts success, south-east is healthful, north enhances love, thus imparts personal progress, whereas north-east forbodes bad luck. Similarly west, south-west and north west direction are also infavourable.

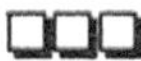

13
Pakwa and Eight Triagrams

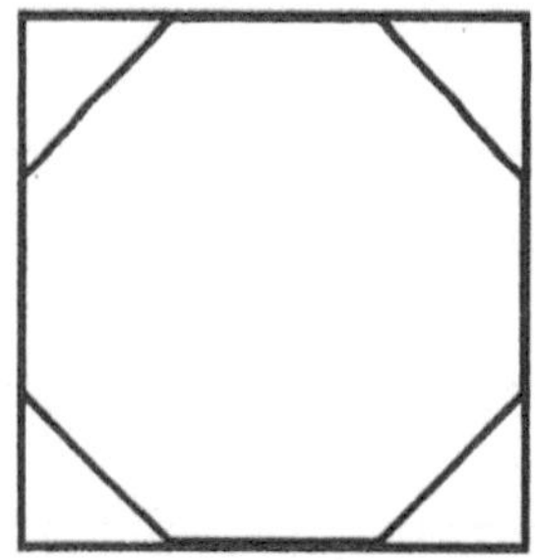

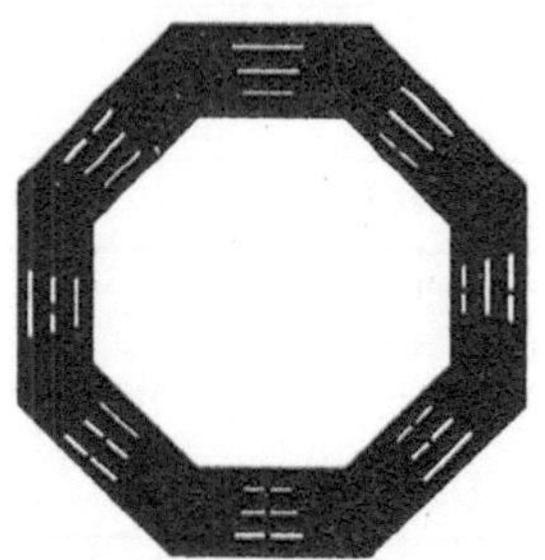

If we draw four transverse lines, that is one line on each of corners of Lo Shui, we will obtain the octagon 'Pa' Kua' which an eight cornered diagram, used in Feng Shui.

In Chinese language 'Pa' means eight and 'Kwa' means a diagram of tree lines. So, Pakwa is an octagonal figure which is a combination of eight specific, Trigrams and octagonal device (Yantra). The Chinese also call this 'compass' , which guides us as to which portion of a house needs 'Chi'.

About 5000 years ago Fu Chi, a Chinese philosopher who was meditating on the bank of the yellow river suddenly realised, that a tortoise had emerged from (out of) the yellow river's water. Fu Chi felt that emergence of a tortoise was God-sent entity on whose back, the map of the entire universe was etched. His serialise description of etching figures or marks on the back of tortoise was called by the name of 'Former Heaven Sequence, A Trigram consists of three lines, and there are eight such diagrams. It is believed that the theories of Yen and Yang and five elements are the very basis of this figure formation. A Trigram is drawn by three lines, which are letter broken or unbroken, Broken and unbroken lines, combined in different configuration, constitute various formations. Which are known as 'Octagonal Diagrams'. The Origin and development of a Trigram is consistent with Yen and Yang lines. Such as,

Yang	Yen
Creation	Heaven

If a line each is added to the above, we obtain the following formations, such as:

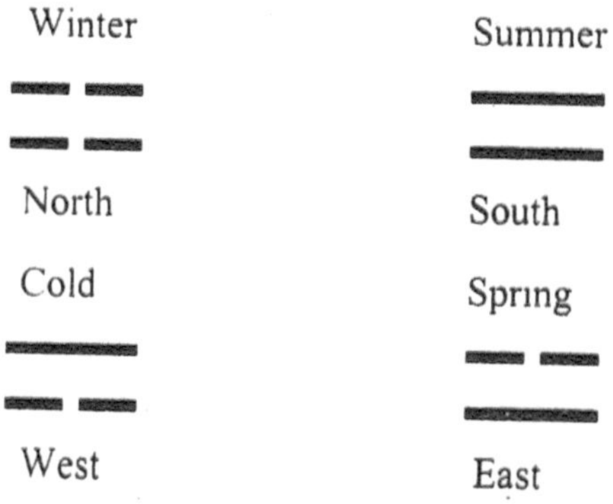

Winter	Summer
North	South
Cold	Spring
West	East

If we add another additional line to the above formations, we will obtain eight Trigrams.

The Chinese have assigned a specific nomenclature to each of the trigrams so as to ensure proper distinction amongst all the Trigrams. Following formations will spell out what we wish to convey.

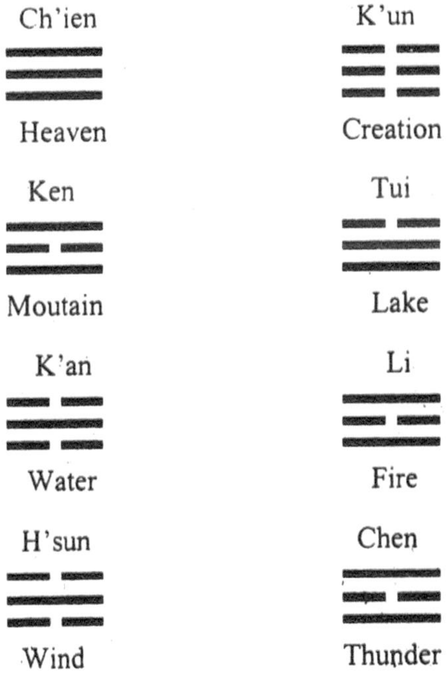

Ch'ien	K'un
Heaven	Creation
Ken	Tui
Moutain	Lake
K'an	Li
Water	Fire
H'sun	Chen
Wind	Thunder

The said Trigrams have been arranged in a sequence which is known as 'Former Heaven Sequence'.

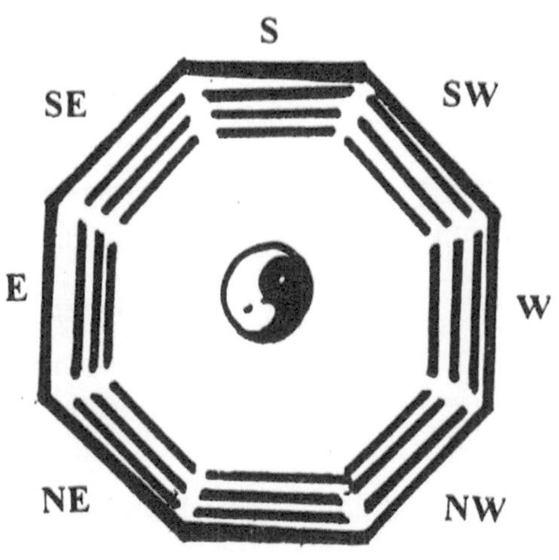

(Former Heaven Sequence)

Emperor Wen and his feudal chief introduced changes in the above octagram, explained the relative details and, thus, created later 'Heaven Sequence. Former Heaven Sequence', was generally used to dispel inimical and wicked 'Sha' and a mirror or Yantra used for the purpose, whereas the compass, which the Chinese navigators used, had 'Later Heaven Sequence' etched on its surface.

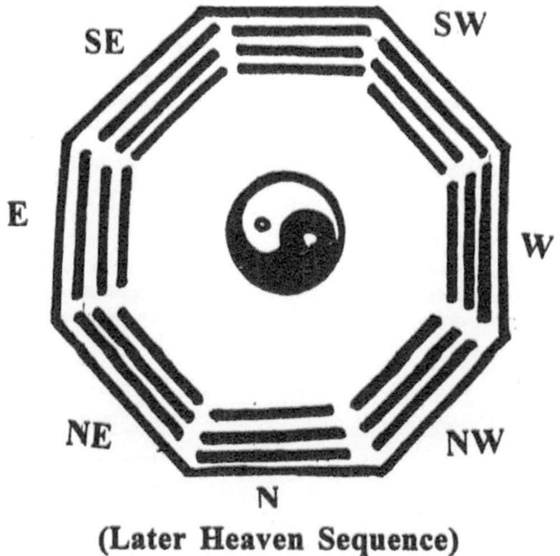

(Later Heaven Sequence)

Unbroken lines denote male sex and these lines are Yang lines, whereas broken lines are Yin lines which denote female sex, three unbroken lines indicates powerful Yang and also denote the father. Three broken lines (☷ ☷) of Kuan indicate optimum concentration of powerful Yen and they are a symbol of mother also.

Li and Ken are two important diagrams, where a broken line exists in between these lines, and it looks as if diving entity. It is through the sun that divine powers descend on earth, which clearly implies that rapport between the divine power and earth is maintained through the sun. According to the Chinese scholars, sun is more potentially powerful in the south direction, hence Li represents this (south) direction.

In Ken an unbroken line is situated between the two broken lines. This Trigram is reverse of the Ken Trigram, hence it represents the northern direction. There exists one unbroken Yen line between the lines which represents female element. It also denotes second daughter who is born

Trigram	Symbol	Element	Person	Tract	Colour	Body	Season	Direction
☰	Heaven	Metal	Father	Scholar	White	Brain	Starting Cold	N.W
☷	Earth	Earth	Mother	Nutrition	Yellow	Stomach		S.W.
☳	Thunder	Wood	Eldest Son		Green	Foot	Spring	East
☵	Water	Water	Second Son	Circle Fear	Black	Ear	Cold	North
☶	• Hill	Earth	Eldest Son	Hurdle	White	Hand	Starting Spring	N.E.
☴	Age	Wood	Eldest Son	Trade Progress	Green	Buttock	Start Summer	S.E.
☲	Fire	Fire	Second daughter	Fire	Red	Eye	Summer	South
☱	Pond	Metal		Mirth	White	Mouth	Cold	West

as a second child. Similarly, that is in between the eldest and the youngest children. In Ken Trigram, there is one broken line which represents manliness, hence Ken indicates birth of the second son. Similarly, all the Trigrams are indicative of specific meaning and peculiarities. The following table will denote representative features, place and peculiar attributes.

There are set out standard yard sticks before each diagram and there are standard norms regarding place, name, traits and representative emblems for each diagram. Three unbroken lines are emblems of 'Chin' which denote a scholarly male and heaven. The three broken lines always represent earth, female and nurturing whenever selection of most suitable land is desired, we should take into account relevant foiled of each Trigram, with respect to its traits and representative factors. For instance, Kitchen should be in the south, dining room in the south west, bed room in the west and all other locations symbol be designated in an accordance with the laid down guidelines. Similarly, selecting of a suitable site for a business premises, sale, production, godown, office and any other place should be according to individual characteristics of the related diagrams.

How to determine direction of a Building or a House

Entrance gate to building plays an important role in respect of prosperity of a land lord. Building should be constructed at such a place where coordination between the building and the environments is possible to establish. The Chinese residents prefer to keep their entrance door (main gate) in the southern direction so that they could benefit from the sun light and also get protection from cold winds and dust raising yellow

Powerful Symbols of Feng Shui

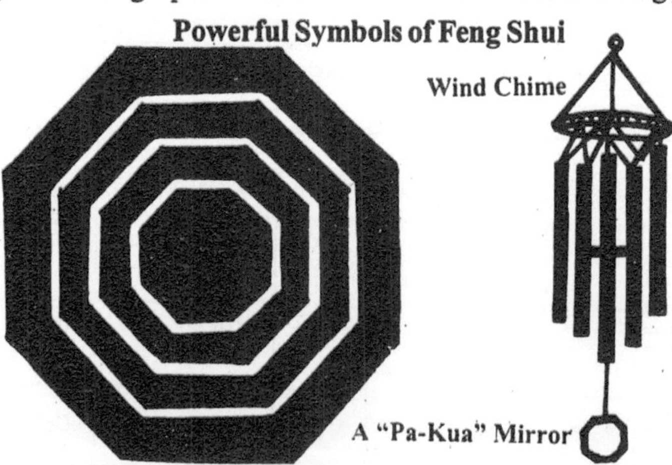

sand. Some do not prefer to keep the main entry door in the north-east and south-west directions, because entry doors on these sides are considered to be doors of devils (evil spirits).

Some Feng Shui scholars determine site and direction of an entry-gate as per year of birth of the head of the family, while others determine, it in accordance with time of birth (as given in the horoscope) of the house-owner. If there are more than one member in a family, then determination of main gate is decided on the basis of horoscope of head of the family. Lo Shu is another method which is employed to determine exact and the most suitable for the main entry-gate.

Keiloon

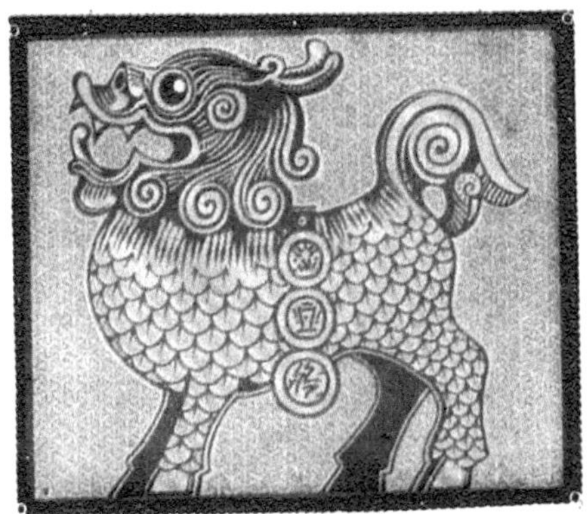

Keiloon is a mythological animal of the Chinese. Its head is like that of a lion and there are also horns on its head. It tail resembles like the tail of a snake, its paws look like hoofs of a goat; hence its name.

There also can be observed three coins on its back. This animal eats thieves, killers and dishonest persons. Its emblem is fixed on the fact so that evil spirits, thieves and dishonest persons are not able to gain entry into a house. If Feng Shui of a house is not in order, then the emblem of this animal should be fixed on the left side of the entrance gate. Keiloon eats unfavourable and harmful powers, for more information, please see another figure of this animal.

Keiloon

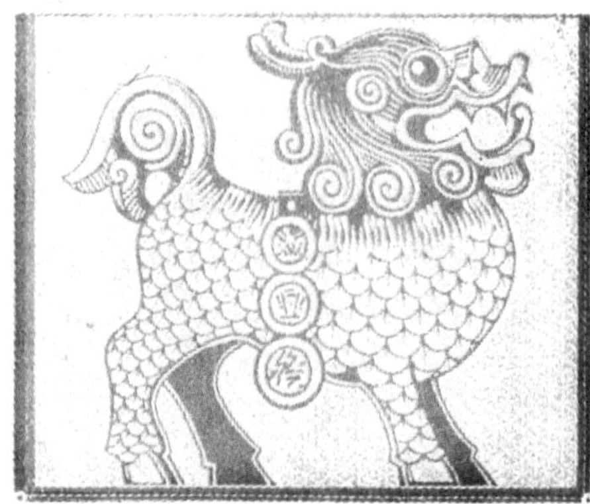

This is a mythological animal of the Chinese whose image or picture is affixed on the right side of an entry gate. Its picture is always affixed in a pair. It serves as a guard to the entry door and keeps away entry of all the inauspicious and harmful objects and elements. In a way it helps to dispel Vaastu related defects and drawbacks, including deficiencies.

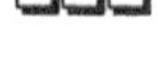

14
Bagua—a symbol of China's ancient architecture

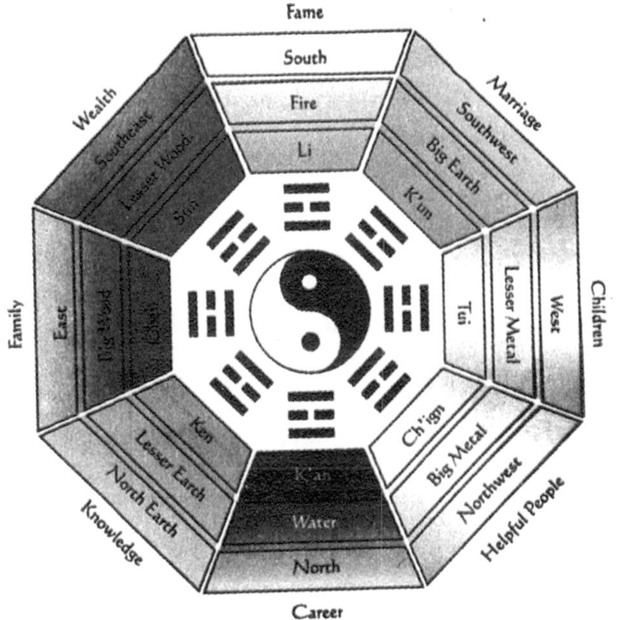

In order to enhance positive changes in life, Bagua is a powerful compass of the Chinese. The talent secret behind its use being that attention should be paid to its peculiar characteristics that be (latently) hidden and use the same with utmost discretion.

Bagua is an octagonal chart. In Chinese language Bagua means a figure 'having eight angles' which signify eight directions. Each point (dot) in the Bagua-compass controls separate facts and phase of life. For instance, facts like knowledge, profession, health, money, fame, marriage, progress and persons who extend help are covered by these points (each point signifying operation of a particular fact) separately. Such facts of life cast their impact upon five elements, caste, weather, figures (numerology) and astronomical life. Tai Chi is situated at the center of Bagua chart which points to Yen and Yang within the circular figure. It is indicative of perfection and reminds that equilibrium is an essential aspect.

It was Fu Shu who established eight Trigrams 5000 years ago, but was established 3000 years ago by emperor Wen and his 'Sammant' (feudal lord) Chou, and the restructured and modified version is known as 'Bagua'. By its utilization, environment can be improved and Chi can be encouraged. It is mainly used to spell out problems that surface during life and also suggest ways and means to solve such problem.

Begua is an octagonal figure which is divided into eight directions, hence it denotes eight conditions of life, as detailed hereunder:-

1. South	Lie,	Fire	Prosperity and fame
2. South-East	H'sien	Wind	Property, wealth and money
3. East	Ch'en	Thunder	Family and health
4. North-East	Ken	Mountain	Knowledge
5. North	K'a	Water	Career
6. North-West	Chien	Heaven	Helping friend.
7. West	Tui	Pond of water	Progeny
8. South-West	Kun	Earth	Marriage.

Relation of Bagua with eight directions

1. South, Li ☲ , Trigram-Fire

Fame, prestige, fortune and festivals are operated through the southern gate. Southern direction has been accorded such a significance by the Chinese and the value it to such an extent that they have kept this season, Red colour, number '9' fire element and also that life is like an imaginative sparrow which never dies. It emerges from the destructive ashes again and again, and forms its body. This is a divine bird that flies high up in the sky, surveys and observes the scenes all around it and then gathers information. It also represents constructivity. This divine birth also imparts inspiration towards deep excitement burning with its celestial beauty. Hence Yen can utilise the salient features of this bird to bring respect to your place of work. You can plan a vast industrial layout, professional details an effective and beneficiary plan for marketing or work out details of budget which will help you to establish your business profession.

In the fire-trigram a broken line exists between the two unbroken lines which induce us to imagine about leaping flames of the fire. Zone of fire elements is indicative of inner light. At any phase or circle of life our conscience gets enlightened by light, rather one should first enlighten his own self (conscience) with the help of light and then enlighten others. When Bagua of a house is strong and powerful, that is the related portion is protruding out, it denotes that the person's fame will enhance and he will attain a respectable position in the society. If, however, Bagua of a house is weak and portion of house or building is missing, then the residents of such a house will be greatly and quickly influenced with the opinion of other persons and he will be having a low self-confidence.

2. South-East Direction (Hasun) ☴, Wind Triagram

Though the dots appearing in a Bagua do invariably, impact wealth and property, in one form or another, yet south-east direction is most potent and powerful direction, which is considered to be a direction related to wealth and property. Perhaps its history can be traced back to business and partnerships that existed between the Chinese and south-east Asian maritime counter parts. The special feature of south-east direction is its number is 4, its colour is considered indigo and the direction ensures pleasure and leisures.

In the wind Trigram there are two unbroken lines and one broken line which denote that wind has immense influence on earth, though its roots are not em bedded in it. Wind is indicative of continuous flow of good fortune and property. Promotion and progress at the place of work, approbation by colleagues and recognition in business are also the attributes of wind element. When the Begua of such a house is powerful, it always yields success in business and excellent fortune. But, if the Bagua of such a house is weak, then it can be the cause of recurring accidents, legal impediments and losses.

3. East (Chen) ☳ , Trigram-Thunder

This direction conducts health, intellect and family life. It represents spring season, green colour and light blue colour, its element being wood, number, and its powerful life force is black snake or a winged snake'. Like a divine power, snake is a far sighted and spiritual enemy. Fast moving of this divine lord gathers various information, contemplates over them and takes intelligent decisions. 'Kaliya' snake is known for its sharp intellect and strength, in Hindu mythology.

This Trigram (Thunder) has two broken and one unbroken lines. Thunder is a powerful force—it rises and then scatters without causing any harm. It presents the elderly which includes (elderly) parents, employers or senior officers. When Bagua of such a house is powerful then a person attains grand success in life. But, if the Bagua is weak, it erodes of working capacity and capabilities.

4. North-East, (Ken) ☶, Trigram-Mountain

Do you wish to widen the basis of your knowledge. Do you want to focus your attention and improve upon concentration, intellectual capabilities? If so, turn to this direction for help. You will find that sea—green colour is active which is a blend of green, and blue colours. Its representative number is '8' which is quite favourable for this direction, and in Chinese language, No '8' is indicative of prosperity.

There are two broken and one unbroken lines in this Mountain-Trigram and it looks like an inner place in a care or a mountain. Mountain is also a symbol of meditation and prayer. If a person persits with (continuous) meditation, he can add to his knowledge. A Bagua house should be well balanced entity. If it is weak, it can be the cause of difficulty in giving birth to children.

5. North (Ken) ☵ ,Trigram-Water

Northern direction conducts profession and success relating to profession. It is one of the most formidable direction which help to surge ahead in a attaining success. Climater of north direction is cold, colour black, basic element water, number is '8' and its animal is tortoise which is considered a symbol of strength, security, permanency and long life. Exact strength of tortoise is on your back from where. It protects your body from attacks. There are two broken and one unbroken lines in the Water-Trigrams, and water is deep in the centre–it is a sign of purity and freedom. Place of water denotes career and it also indicates an unhindered passage of life, apart from capacity to take decisions independently. When the Bagua of a house is powerful, it indicates that the dweller in the house will get money and he will make use of this money for a better cause. But, when Bagua of this house is not powerful, it denotes that some member in the family will fall sick.

6. North-West (Chien)☰ , Heaven Trigram

If far-off places attract you and your tendency is such that distracts you or takes you away from family atmosphere, then strengthen and nurture the north-west portion of your life. If you wish to expand your business outside your city or say you wish to impart a national or international status to it, north-west corner of your office should be extended through guidance of a Feng Shui expert. If Bagua of a house is strong, then the person living in such a house is highly liberal and he helps economically weaker person but if Bagua of a house is debilitated, then such a person will remain tormented by his employees.

7. West (Tui) ☱, Trigram-Lake or Pond

Western direction conducts progeny, fortune of progeny, happiness and constructivity. Its season is autumn, colour white, basic element metal. Number '7' and animal being a ferocious and dreadful Tiger or a Lion. At times a powerful and dreadful animal like Tiger could also prove to bet the best saviours and defenders. As a tiger is always alert and remains warned and guarded against imminent danger. But if this animal is not carefully, controlled, he can suddenly prove dangerous also. In fact, lion or tiger element represents sudden emergence of violence in human character. But, the lion is well controlled, he can prove to be your best friend whenever you desire to hit upon any novel plan.

In a lake Trigram a broken line is placed over two unbroken lines which resembles an open space in the raised surface and a deep lake in the lower surface. A lake-house represents construction functions. It also helps in case of progeny, planning, art and new zeal in life. When Bagua of a house is powerful, then the person is happy and leads excellent life. But, when Bagua of a house is weak, the (same) persòn finds it quite and onerous task to accumulate money even for this happiness and comfort.

8. South-West (Kun) ☷, Trigram : earth

South-west direction of the compass conducts relations, marriage, partnership and maternal love. If you are in search of a suitable partner in business or to strengthen any business relation further, you should make this region more active. South-west direction's colour is yellow, Number '2' and its basic element is sand (of the earth).

The Earth-Trigram is made up of three unbroken lines. It is such a positive power that it spells out necessary principles for a happy marriage. If Bagua of a house is powerful, the female inmates of the house are happier that their male counterparts. But if Bagua of a house is weak, such females may have to face difficulties of various types. It is also a representative of land and agriculture related problems.

Uses and Advantages of Bagua

Since Bagua is shaped as an octagonal figure, it can be easily superimposed to assess position of a plot of land, a room or furniture. If there are impediments in married life, there are problems about progeny, when someone has no child, then Bagua should be superimposed in the house and thus one can find out weak or strong position of Bagua (and also the reasons therefore) in relation to directions. One's fortune can be improved as the discerned defects are removed. Procedure to implement Bagua is quite simple. The method, which is employed to correctly install Bagua, is called by the name of the 'Three doors of Chu'. It is necessary to understand position of the main-gate of a house, before using Bagua, and there should be no confusion in this regard. Main entrance gate is that part of the house from where energy flows. In foreign countries, front door of the house is kept shut and movement (entry and exit) is affected through the back-door. Hence back door is given more importance in this case.

When Bagua is used for a house or a portion of the house, then the main door becomes most important. If the door is situated in the middle it denotes career and a door on the right side denotes helpful friends, while a door on the left is an emblem of knowledge. Each door in the house creates different Baguas. For example, a door at a boundary wall, main gate of the house, door of the drawing room, and door of the retiring room has its own individual Bagua.

Every storey in a multistoried building creates its individual Bagua that is each storey has its own Bagua that differs from Bagua of other storeys.

According to Feng Shui, Bagua of a storey will start from the place where the stairs to that story end, and its field of activity will also remain confined to all the rooms situated in that storey. Bagua is also used in the case of plots of irregular size, and also to establish coordination among rooms.

The Feng Shui experts can quite easily find out the trouble spots and problem ridden sites in a house with the help of Bagua. A plot or house of an unusual dimension/detineates defects of the area, in relation to the house. If a plot or house is not shaped square or rectangular, then some part of it will be protruding out or will be found missing. The former position will be called 'Positive area' and the later one as a 'Negative area' but, if half or more than half portion of a plot is protruding either width or length wise, then it will be termed as a 'Negative area'. If the providing portion is less than half the dimension of length, then it will remain a 'Positive area'.

A house or room can be made favourable if principles of Bagua are applied. For instance, if an area of property is 'extinct or missing' in a building or room, then resident in such places may have to face financial problems. But such a defect can be warded off by a mirror, plants or crystal back in the extinct area, by adhering to principles explained for Bagua, it will remove the defects and eliminate deficiencies, thereby adding to the luck of the place. Similarly, if a flower pot or a red rose is kept in any office it may ensure popularity. Vaastu related faults can be remedied by using anyone of the remedial devices liked mirror, light, plants, transparent ball of glass (say crystal ball), bells, flute, use of colours etc. If these devices are used, as per requirement, that will enhance happiness and prosperity.

"Pa-Kua" Model

The indispensable energetic overlay of Feng Shui

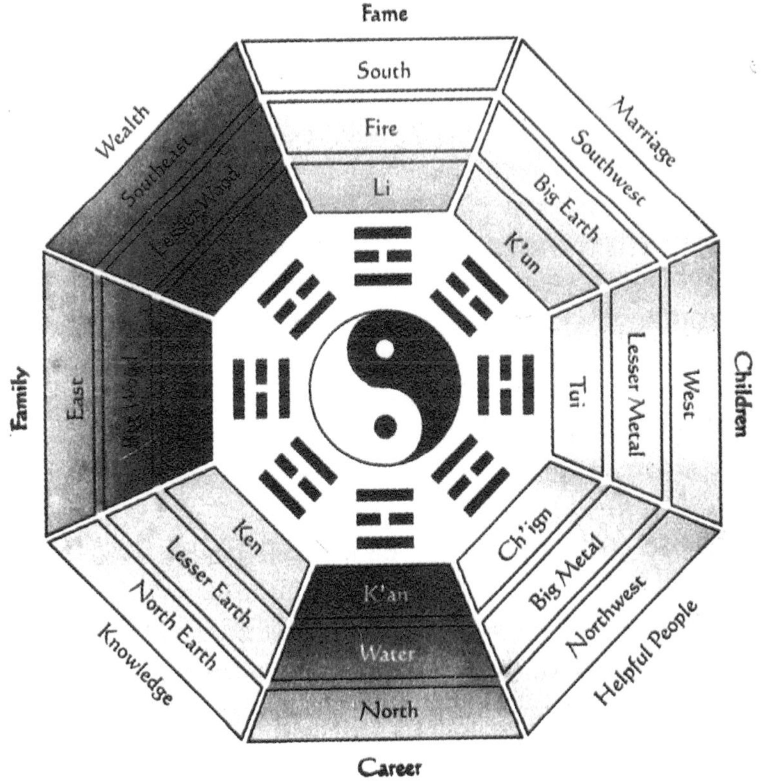

15
Door-Planning through Pa-Tzu Method

Pa-Tzu is an ancient Chinese method to determine lucky and favourable directions of a house. Pa-Tzu is based on eight Trigrams and Lo Shu Picture. It not only points to the most favourable side, but also indicates favourable and unfavourable areas. Method of calculation is the same as explained earlier, with reference to Lo-Shu method. After knowing your annual number, You can also know about element and suitable and favourable colours.

Pa-Tzu method has been divided into two parts. First part pertains to eastern zone and the second to western zone. Eastern zone also includes north-east, south-west and southern directions. Similarly, western zone also includes north-east, north-west, west and south-west directions. If your annual number is 1,3,4 or 9 then north, east, south-east and southern directions will be lucky for you. If your animal number comes to 2,6,7 or 8 then south-east, north-west, west and south-west directions will prove lucky for you. If in calculation, your annual number comes to 5, it will be reckoned as No. '2' for males and No. '8' for females.

Illustration

If a person is born in 1949, men's annual number will be '6' and women's will be '9'. So lucky direction for the males will be north-east, north-west and south-west. Similarly, for the females born during this year north-east, south-east and southern directions will be lucky. Hence, if they keep the main gate in the north or east direction, and bedroom in the south direction, it will prove favourable for them.

Beneficial Directon for Men	S	NE	W	NW	SW	SE	E	SW	N
Year Number of Men	9	8	7	6	5	4	3	2	1
Birth Year	1901	1902	1903	1904	1905	1906	1907	1908	1909
	1910	1911	1912	1913	1914	1915	1916	1917	1918
	1919	1920	1921	1922	1923	1924	1925	1926	1927
	1928	1929	1930	1931	1932	1933	1934	1935	1936
	1937	1938	1939	1940	1941	1942	1943	1944	1945
	1946	1947	1948	1949	1950	1951	1952	1953	1954
	1955	1956	1957	1958	1959	1960	1961	1962	1963
	1964	1965	1966	1967	1968	1969	1970	1971	1972
	1973	1974	1975	1976	1977	1978	1979	1980	1981
	1982	1983	1984	1985	1986	1987	1988	1989	1990
	1991	1992	1993	1994	1995	1996	1997	1998	1999
Year Number of Women	6	7	8	9	1	2	3	4	5
Beneficial Direction for Women	NW	W	NE	S	N	SW	E	SE	NW

In this chart, in the upper part the suitable direction for men and in the lower part suitable direction for women have been mentioned. For example a man born in 1967 has number 6 and north-west direction as suitable for him, while for women born in the same year number 9 and south as the suitable direction have been mentioned.

West

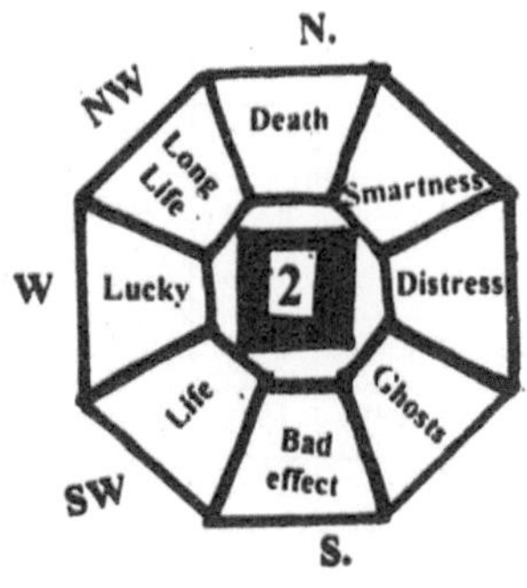

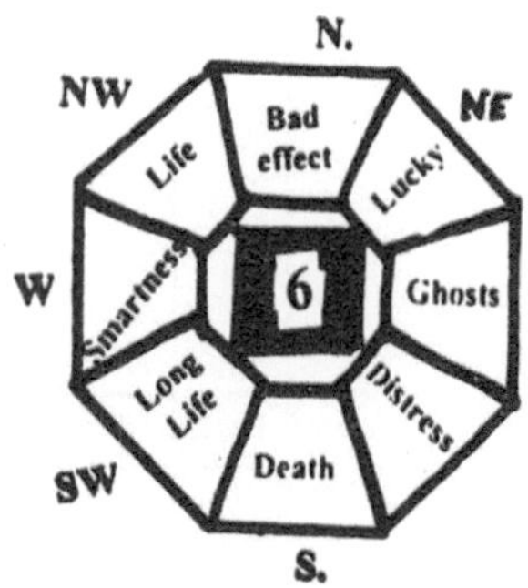

Element—Earth
Colour—Yellow

Element—Metal
Colour—White

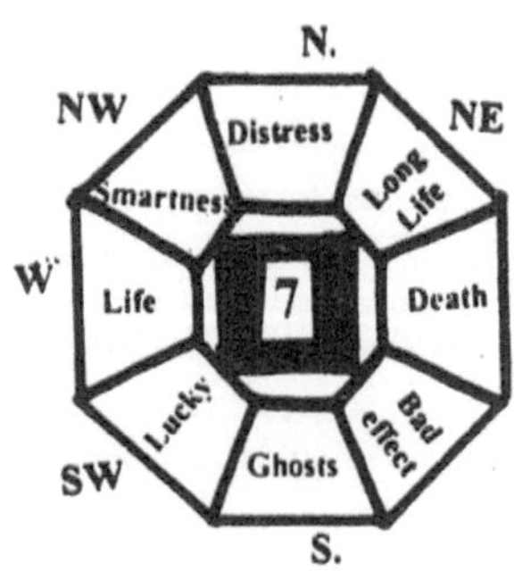

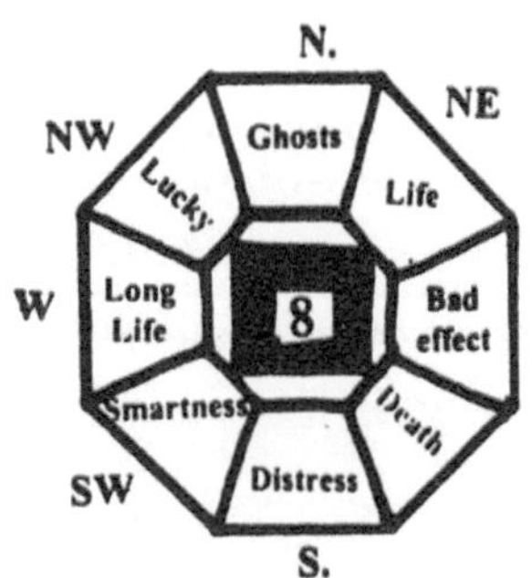

Element—Metal
Colour—White

Element—Earth
Colour—Yellow

East

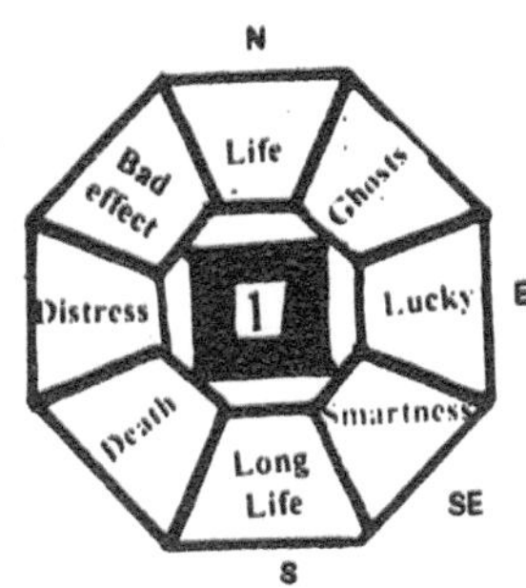

Element—Water
Colour—Black

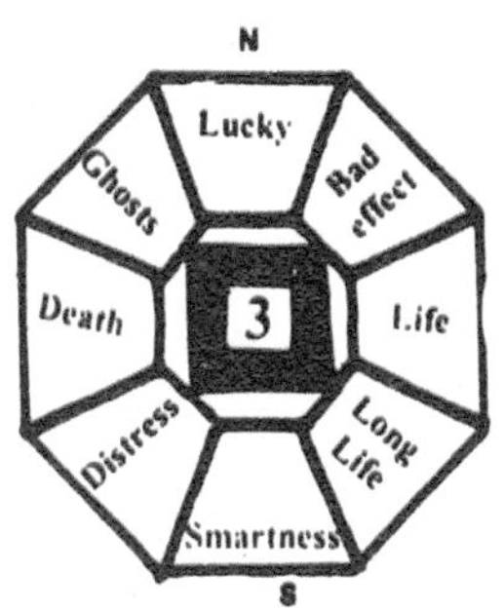

Element—Wood
Colour—Green

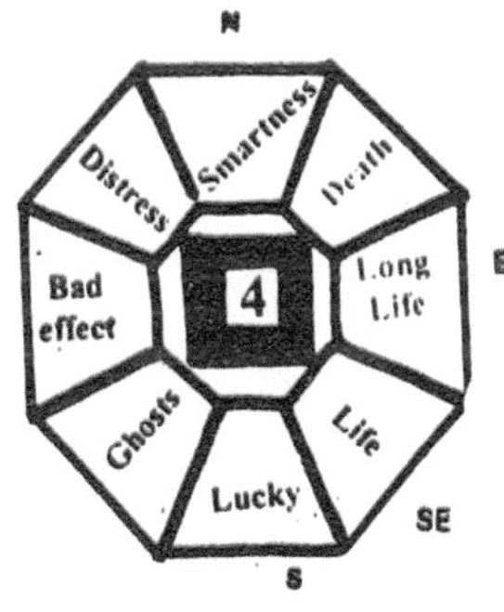

Element—Wood
Colour—Green

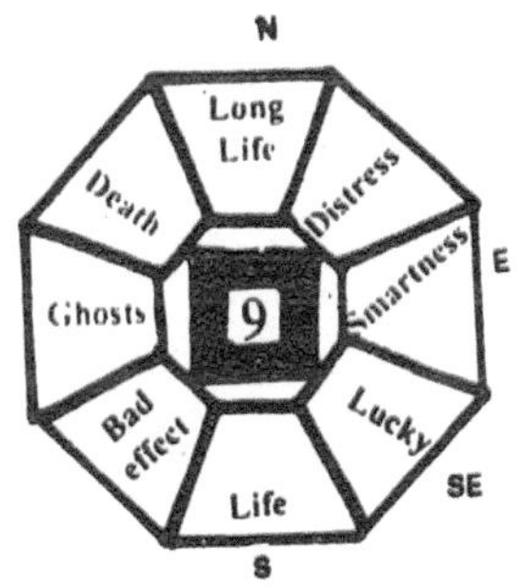

Element—Fire
Colour—Red

❑❑

16
Lou Pan Compass

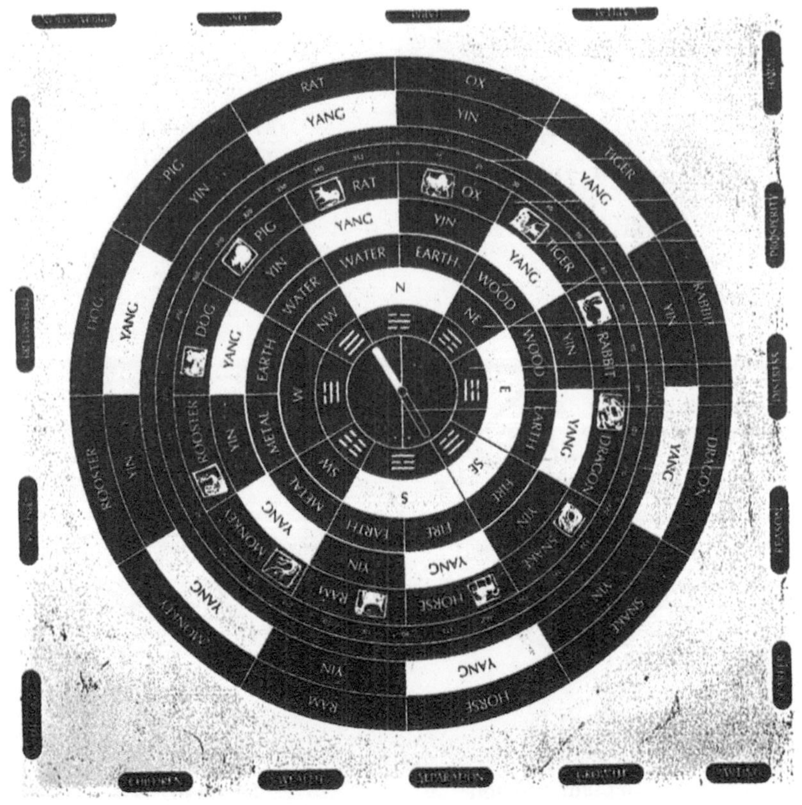

A "Luo Pan"
The essential Feng Shui reference compass

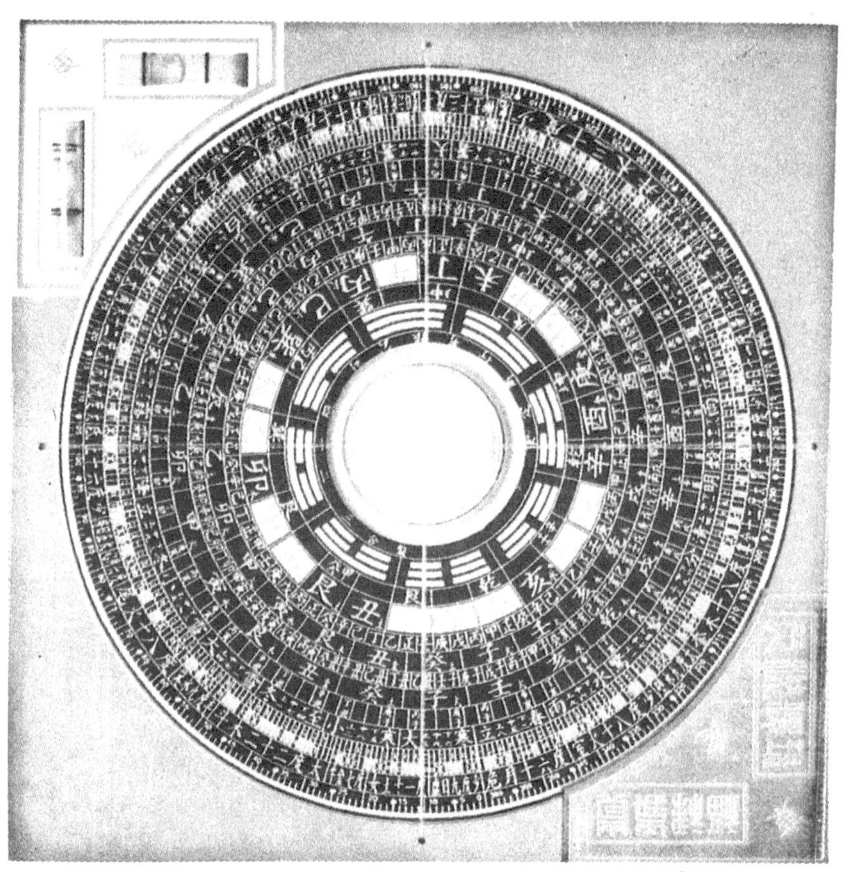

❑❑❑

17
Selection of a bed according to Five Elements

1. Earth Element and Wood Element

Professional

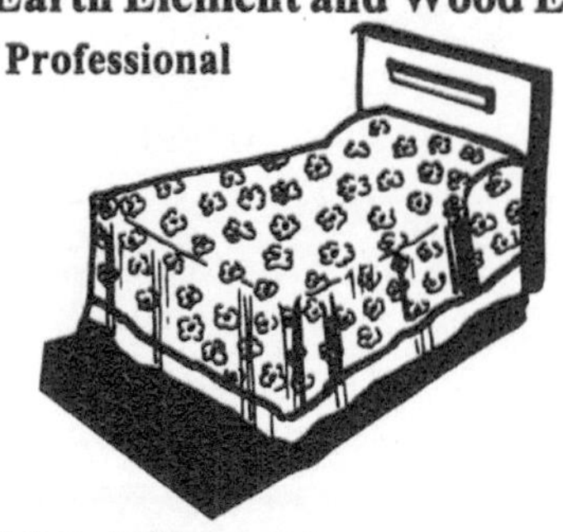

1. Square shaped pillow represents earth and wood elements, hence such a type of pillow is useful for persons born in earth and wood elements, and also useful for those who are professionals.

2. Metal Element

Trader Labourer

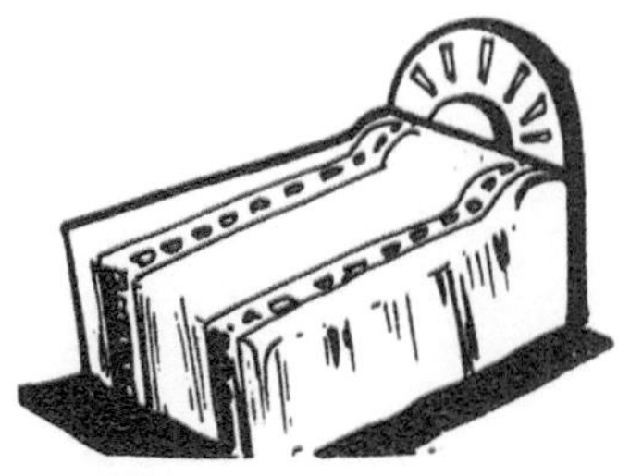

2. A half-moon shaped or a round bed Half-moon or wind shaped beds are considered useful for the persons working in factories, workshops, paper mills etc. because such beds denotes metal element. Hence, for the persons whose element is metal or those who work in factories/workshops, such type of bed creates excellent Feng shui.

3. Fire Element

Meant for those who do not wish to sleep

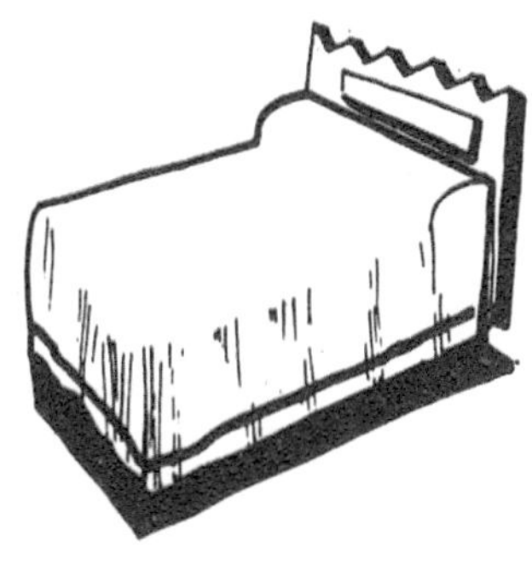

3. A bed having triangular shape at the head-side are inauspicious because it is dominated by fire element, will disturb sleep.

4. Water Element

Art lover, Musician

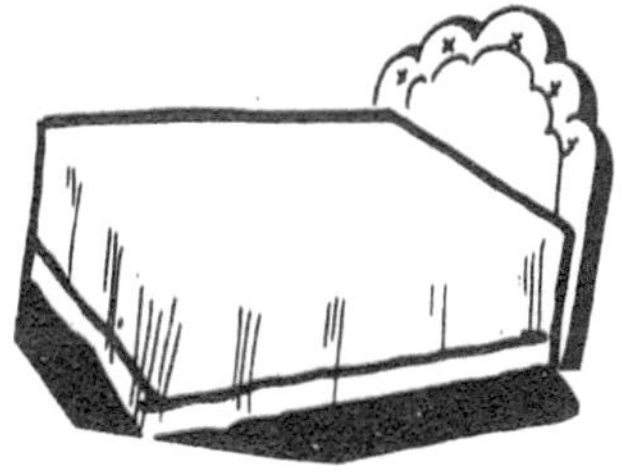

4. A wary type of bed denotes water element. It is an ideal bed for persons born in water elements and artists, music lover and engineers.

❑❑❑

18
Feng Shui Rules for Bed-rooms

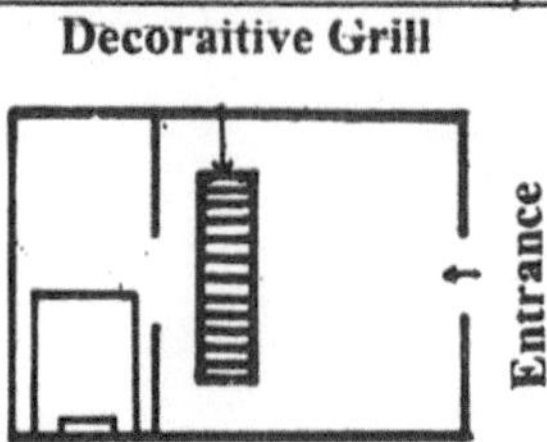

1. There should be no direct entry from the main entrance door to your bed-rooms. There ought to be a partition or decorative mesh between the main door and bedroom. According to rules of Feng Shui, if there is direct entry from the main gate to the bedroom, the owner of the house will remain emblamed in litigation and will also be mentally tense. Hence the bedroom of a person should be a secret place where there is privacy.

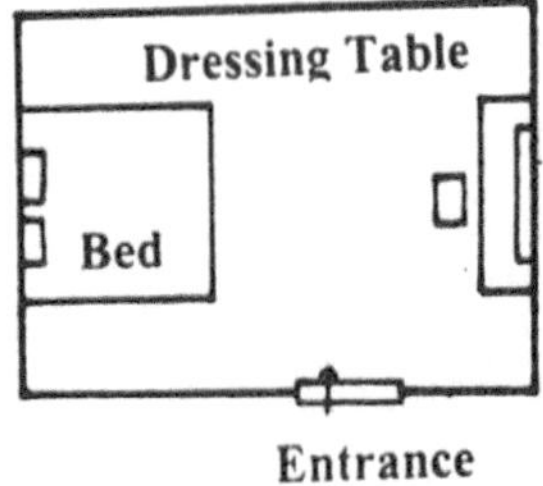

2. Similarly, dressing table should not be placed in front of your bed's head-side. It often occurs that a person gets scared if he sees his

own image in the mirror, when he gets up during sleep.

According to Feng Shui, the person concerned will be embroiled with multiple problems due to unknown reason. If dressing table is placed in front of the head side. As a rule, there should be no dressing-table in the bed-room. But if, at all it is necessary, it should be kept on the left or right side of the bed.

3. Also do not keep any picture, showing water, or an aquarium in the bed-room.

Rules regarding sleeping in the bed

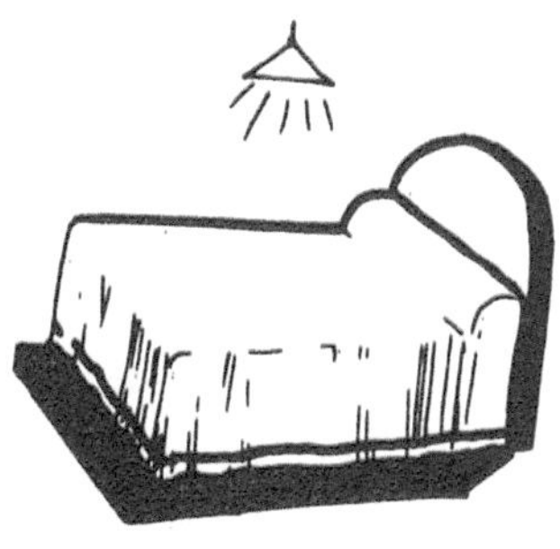

4. Bed should be cosy and comfortable, but there should be no light over the bed nor electric device like fan, lamp etc. otherwise the digestive capacity of the person sleeping will get weakened.
5. Similarly, never keep any watch under your pillow or beneath the bed, nor even in your front, otherwise you will remain worried. For the best Feng Shui watch should be kept on the right or left side of your bed.
6. Keeping pillow and bed-sheet of simple design on the bed.

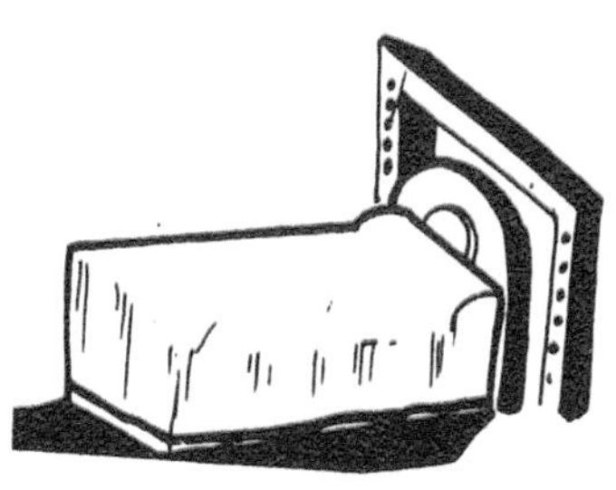

19
Type of doors according to Five elements

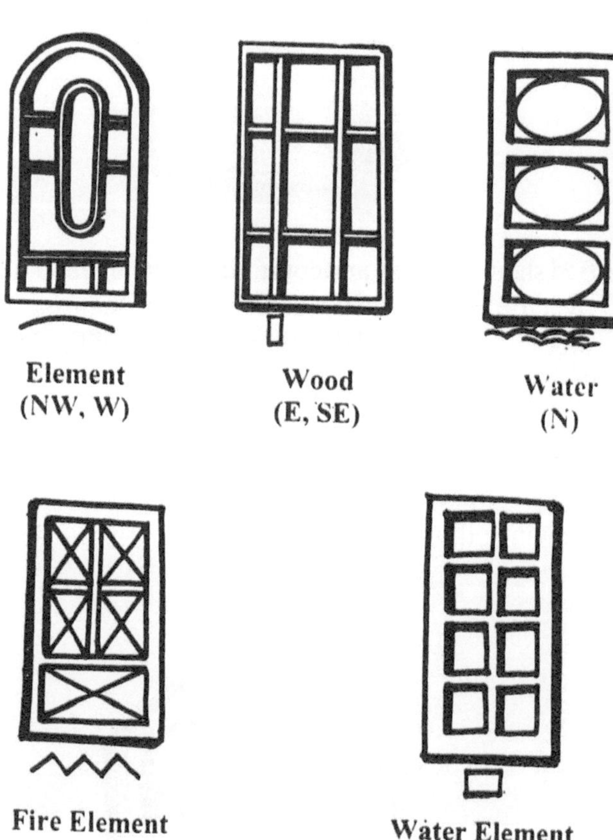

Element
(NW, W)

Wood
(E, SE)

Water
(N)

Fire Element

Water Element

Windows on both sides of the main entrance gate

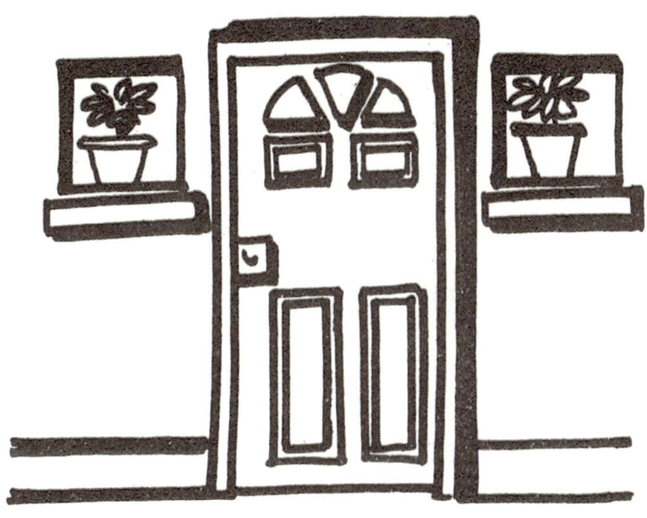

In Feng Shui it is an ominous sign of windows exist on both sides of the main gate, because it will expose the safety of your house, so that winds from both the side will destroy the positive energy 'Chi', resulting in financial disparities for the house-owner.

Remedy

Grow or keep plants of round leaves on both the windows, but do not plant or use cactus and plants having sharped/conical leaves.

Here money-plant is more suitable.

Tree in front of main entrance door of a house

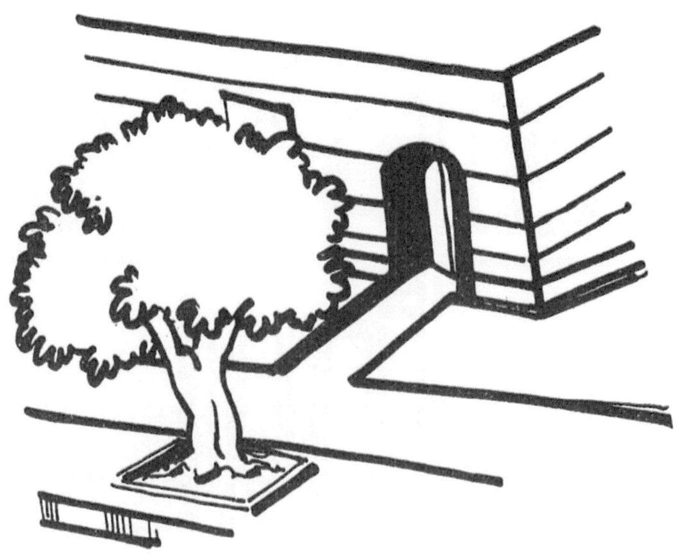

Existence of any tree in front of the main entrance door is an ominous sign in Feng Shui. Its impact will result in the form of illness to the house owner, who will remain troubled due to unwanted problems and court cases.

Remedy

Dangle octangonal mirror outside the main entrance door-it will dispel negative energy and, thus, will not let it enter the house.

Main gate obstructed by stocking of building material or a built-up house (in front of the house)

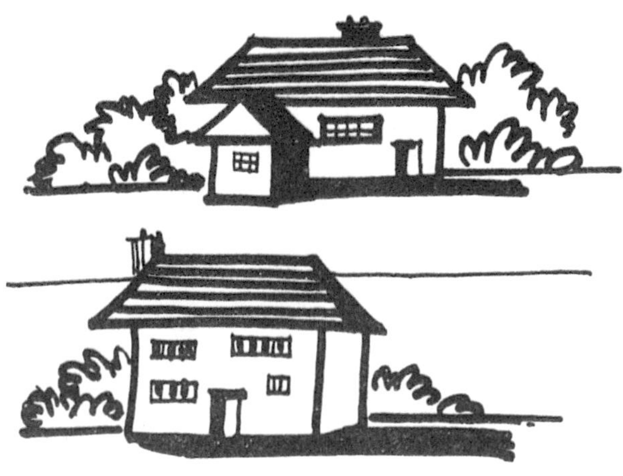

It is an inauspicious sign in Feng Shui if main gate gets blocked or obstructed due to stocking of building material or construction work for a house, or an already built-up house-it can cause heart-attack to the house-owner. Similarly, if corner of another house obstructs main gate of the house, even the house owner can suffer from heart disease.

Remedy

Dig earth at the main entrance, then place six golden coins underneath or dangle an octangonal mirror outside the main gate.

Main Gate of a house situated in front of a lift (Elevator)

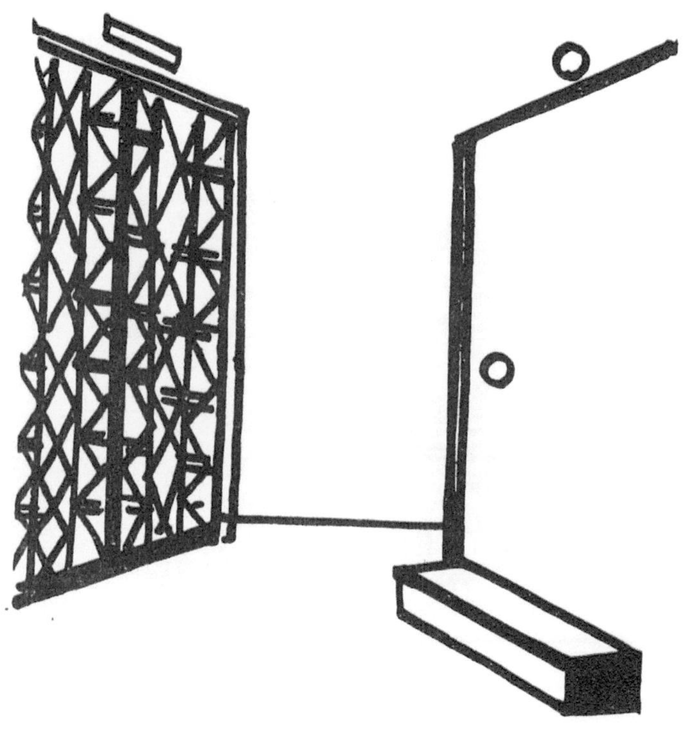

Existence of an elevator (lift) in front of your house or flat is considered an ominous sign in Feng Shui. As the door of the lift opens and shuts every now and then, it causes an adverse impact on the fortune of the house-owner.

Remedy

Dangle an octangonal mirror above the main entrance gate and also raise level of the threshold by 2 inches from the ground level.

If a main door exists above the stairs

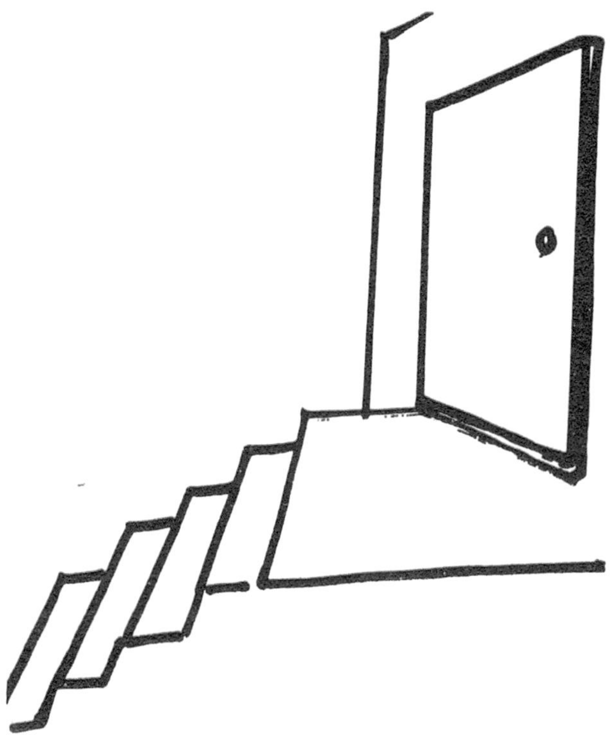

If you have to scale some stairs first in order to reach the main gate of a house or flat, that if the main gate exists where the last stair ends, it is not considered an auspicious sign in Feng Shui. In such a situation, wealth and prosperity will slide down and pass out through the stairs, and the house-owner will not be able to reap the fruits of this hardwork.

Remedy

Hang (dangle) an octagonal mirror over the main entrance gate.

Main door in front of the stairs

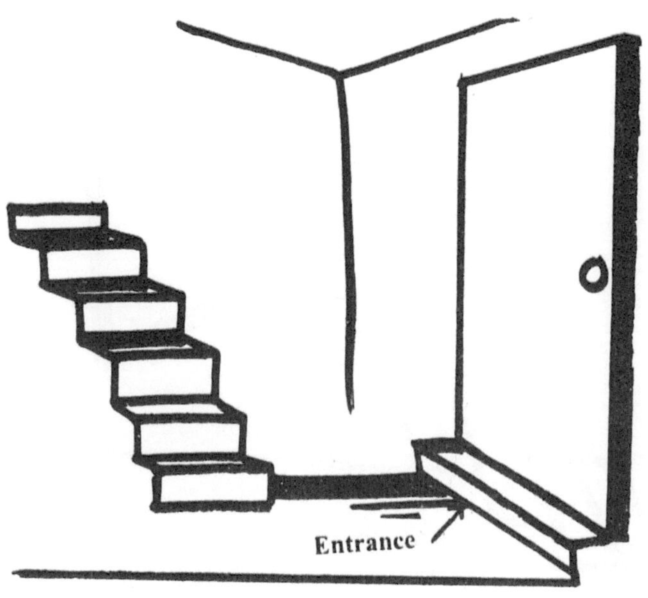

If the main entrance gate of your house or flat is positioned in front of the stairs, it is also an ominous sign according to Feng Shui. The owner of such a house or flat will remain in disposed and strength of his body will also wane.

Remedy

Ominous impact caused by the said position of main door and stairs can be rectified if plinth of the hildreth is elevated to a minimum height of two inches.

Three doors in a straight line

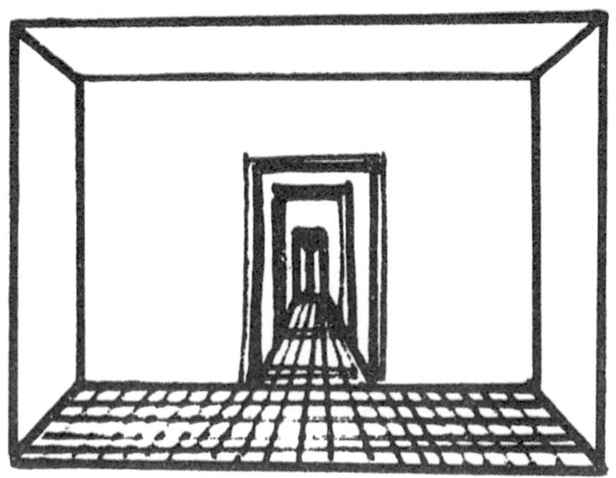

According to Feng Shui if three doors are positioned in a row-that one door is followed by another door on its backside, it results in quick exist of positive energy 'Chi' through these doors. As a rule such positive energy should always enter in a house through the main door. If that does not happen, failing in which prosperity will be uncertain.

Remedy

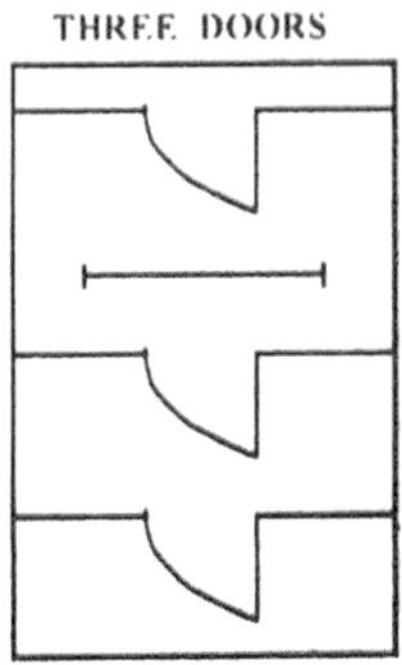

In order to offset the damaging impact, caused by existence of 'Chi' energy, paint/dangle a decorative window (as is done by the furniture makers) on the second door (next to and behind the main door). It is better the last door is kept closed for most of the time. Window painting should be as mentioned hereunder.

20
Positions of Desk or Table according to Feng Shui

Wrong position

The desk where you sit and the table whereon you work should be kept at an appropriate place because your career and future are directly related to wrong position of desk or table.

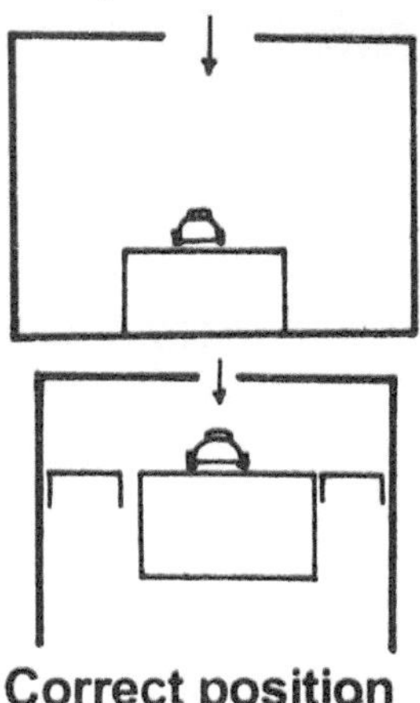

Correct position

1. If your desk is positioned in front of a door and your back is towards the the gate, it is absolutely an incorrect and harmful position.
2. Even sitting or placing the desk in the immediate proximity to the gate is also wrong. In both the situations the house-owners will be ditched, his decisions will be wrong and he will not be able to concentrate his mind, hence avoid such situations.

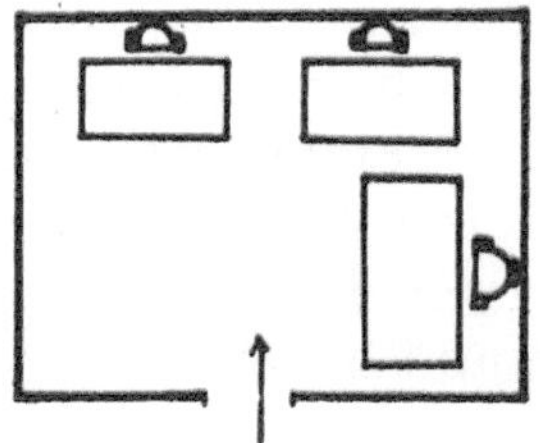

According to Feng Shui directions, you should keep your back towards the wall and keep your eyes towards the gate. All the three positions shown in diagram No. 3, are correct and ideal positions. Correct direction is also a significant

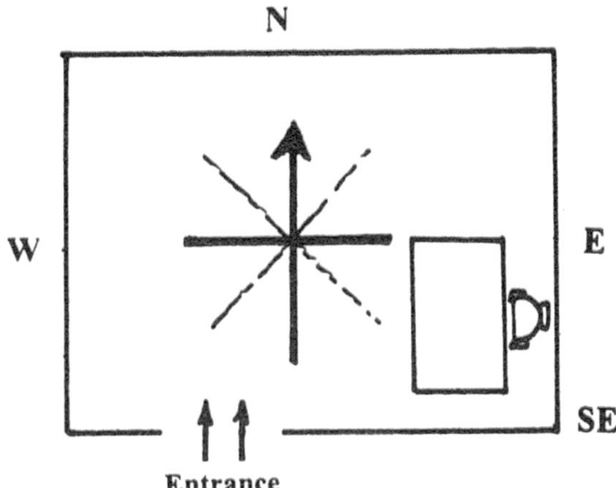

factor, hence direction should also be idealy situated; because your success depends on this eastern or north-eastern direction.

❑❑❑

21
Position of Houses according to Feng Shui

House situated at 'S' corner

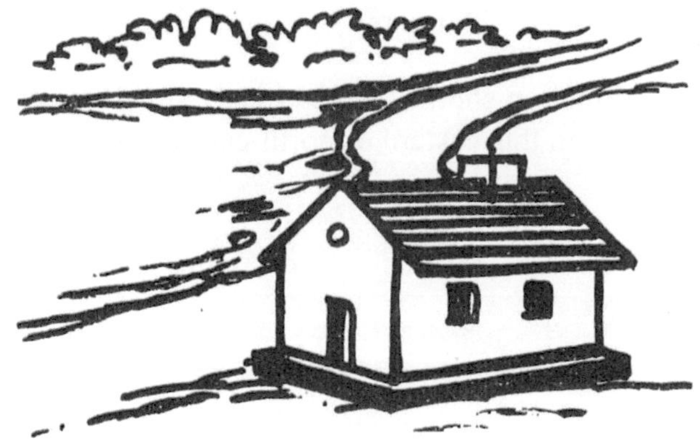

It is an excellent Feng Shui position, if a house is situated at the corner of "South" as it bestows property, wealth and prosperity on the house owner. While purchasing a new house, the following points may be kept in mind, viz.

1. ***Sun light must freely enter into the house.***
2. ***Natural wind should enter into the house.***
3. ***Do not purchase a house, if it is owned by a person who continues to face failures.***
4. ***Do not purchase a house or flat at the top-most floor.***
5. ***Do not purchase any house in whose vicinity a hospital, burial ground or a church exists, or if any one of these places exists in front of the house.***
6. ***Do not purchase a house whose curvature is obleguity or has many corners.***

If a house is situated on the corner of an 'L' shaped Road

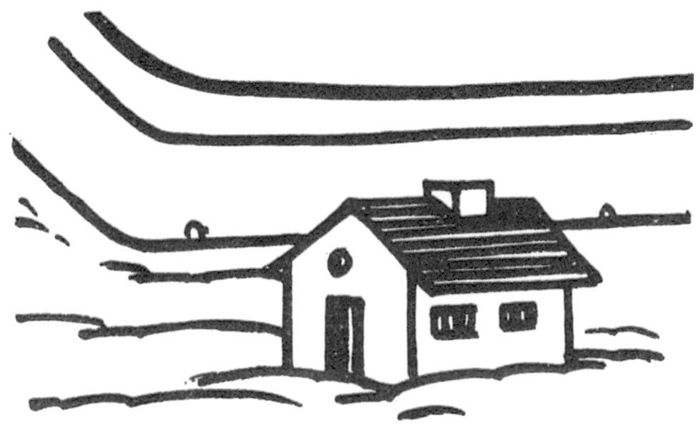

If a house situated at the corner of an 'L-shaped' road and is also situated one the right side of the road (as shown in above diagram), such a house is termed as a house built on knife's cut. According to Feng Shui the owner of such a house will continue to face problems on account of luck and money, and both will be faced with many bottlenecks. Moreover, he will reel under the fear of meeting with some accident.

Remedy

Do not erect the main entrance gate in the middle portion of the house, but only in the corner of the house. Erect small fencing outside the main gate and dangle an octangle mirror on the wall which faces the road.

A house situated outside a half-moon Shaped circle

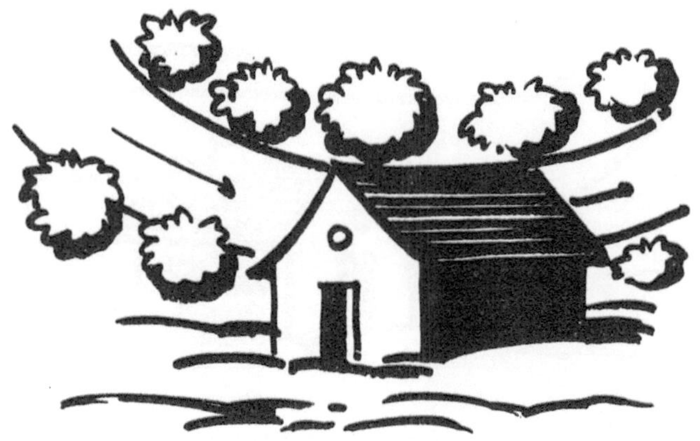

If any house falls outside the ambit of a half-moon shaped circle (as shown in the above figure), the dwellers in such a house will face economic difficulties. According to Feng Shui they will also face continuous ups and downs in life. Morever, these residents will perform such acts the fruit of which they have to face in the form of losses, that is they will themselves be the cause of their losses.

Remedy

Plant bushes around the main entry door and also within the circle where the half-moon is formed.

If a house is situated within the semi-circle

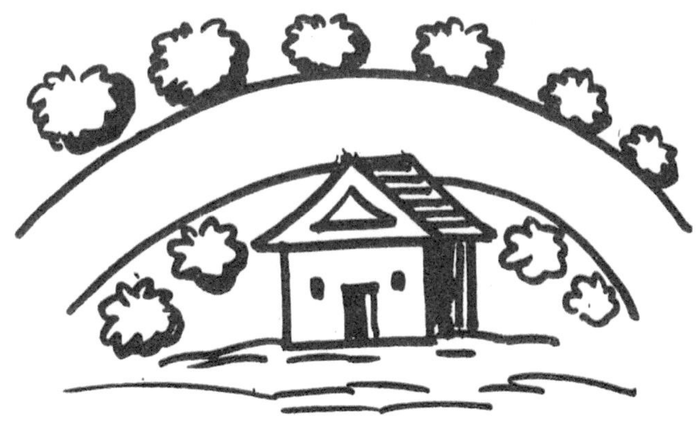

If a house is situated within the ambit of half-moon shaped circle, it is an excellent situation according to Feng Shui.

If two highways converge towards a house in a 'V' Shape

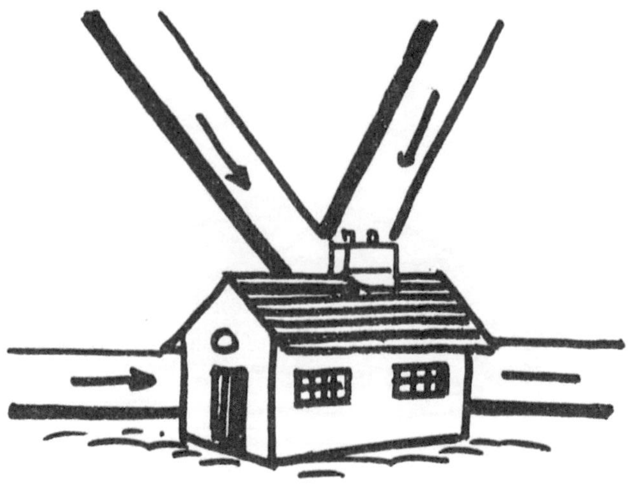

If two highways converge in a 'V'-Shape towards a house, it is considered an ominous sign in Feng-Shui, as both the men and women leaving in such a house, will remain ill and their monetary position will also be weak

Remedy

Erect a door in the house but keep it away from the converging point of 'V' -Shaped highways. Fix a mirror in the door facing the highways erect a small boundary wall around the house, or plant mini plants or bushes so that they look like a boundary wall, so that negative energy can not enter the house directly. If there are two doors in the house, both should not be opened simultaneously.

A highway that intersects a house from two sides

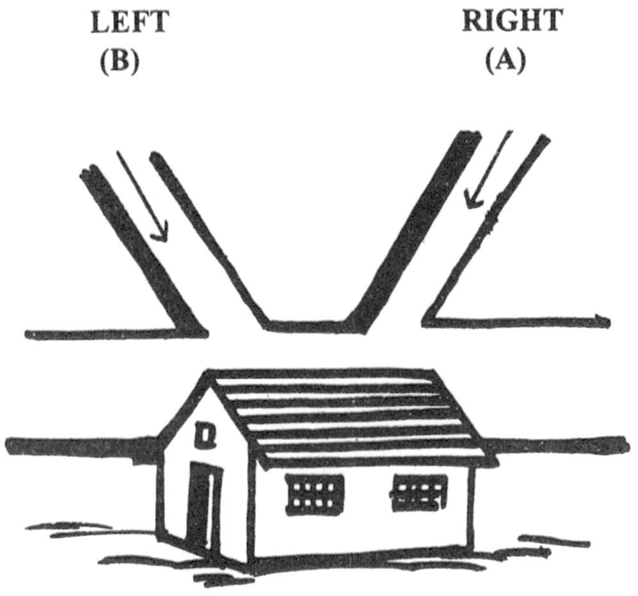

If path of a national high way intersects a house from two corners and also proceeds towards it, is not auspicious situation according to Feng Shui, because money disappears from such a house quickly. If the road proceeds towards a house from the right side (also called the figure side), lady of such a house might meet accidents or may fall prey to fear psychosis, caused by some impending or suspected mishap.

Remedy

Fix the door in such a way that it should look to have been fixed at a corner. Dangle an ordinary mirror or an octagonal mirror on the wall that faces the road.

A vacant place or garden in the back yard of a house

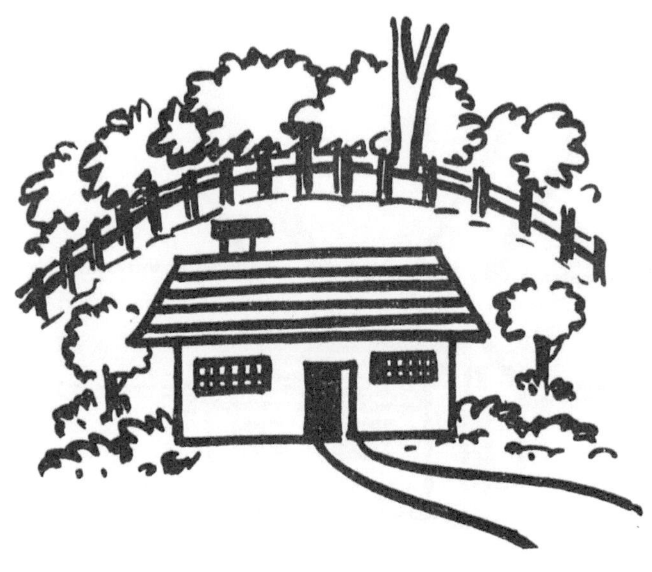

If there is a vacant place or a garden on the back side of a house, but not a big house or mountain or plateau exists, it is not considered a good situation in Feng Shui. Such a house is unsafe as positive energy 'Chi' will waste away, as it will disappear or exit through the back side.

Remedy

Construct a boundary wall between the vacant area or garden, or plant large sized trees in a row so that positive energy remains within the boundary wall—it will keep the house energised by the 'Chi' energy.

A house situated at the'T'-junction

Negative forces will be active in a house situated at a T-junction (See the figure). According to Feng Shui, health of head of the family remains a constant cause of worry for the family members, because any mishap could occur at any time.

Remedy

If possible shift the main door from the centre of the road to a corner. The main entrance gate should have two or three doors. Keep the central door shut, and entry should be from the side door/doors. Place an octagonal mirror outside the main gate of the house.

A house having multiple windows

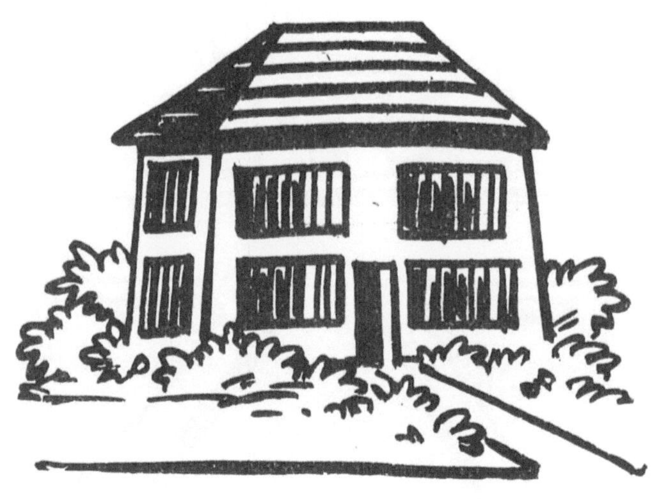

If there exist many windows and doors all around a house, then excessive wind and light will be let in that house, and it will result in excess storage of Yang energy. The winds blowing through the windows will get blended so as to impede free flow of 'Chi', as a result of which the house-owner will become peevish and snobbish, and he will have loss of patience also.

Remedy

Keep some of the windows closed. Use curtains on the windows so that entry of light could be restricted to some extent.

Do not watch a laundry from window of house

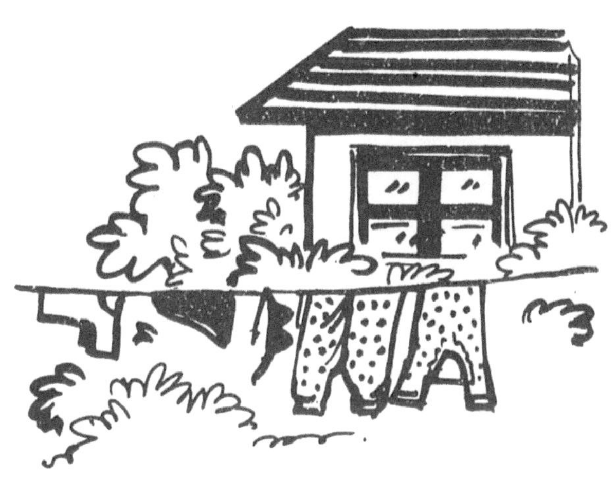

It is harmful if a neighbour's garden, laundry place, washing machine or wet clothes are seen from the window of a house. According to Feng Shui, if the distance from, the window is within 30-100 metres and also when ladies underwears, vests, bras and gowns are seen, it adversely impacts 'Yin' energy that it adds to Yin's ill effects, due to which the house-owner will always feel the paucity of money and the earned money will slip away from his hands.

Remedy

Hang curtains on both sides of the window (s) and have control over wasteful expenses.

Satellite or dish antenna in front of the main door or main windows of the house

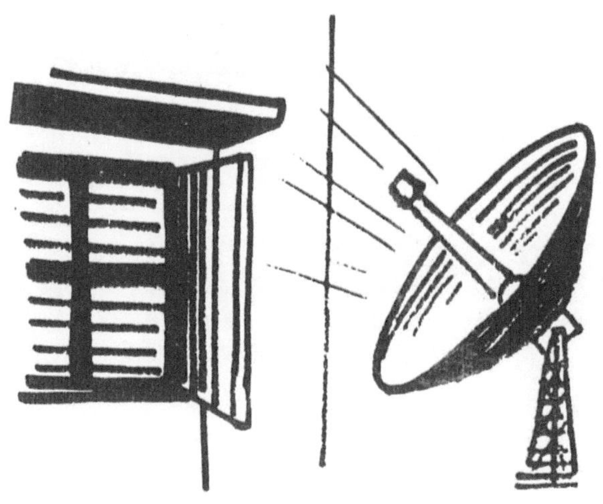

If a satellite or dish antenna is situated in front of the main door or window. It destroys 'Chi' the positive energy in the house, according to Feng Shui.

Remedy

Fix a net (mesh) or hang a curtain before the main door and grow good plants in a flower pot (of clay) outside the main windows so that the positive energy 'Chi' does not get destroyed.

If a highway exists at the back side of the house

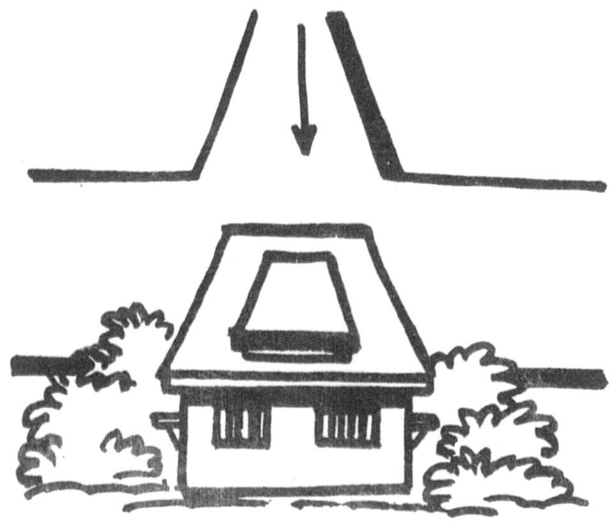

If a road exists at the back side of the house, You should think someone is stabbing you in the back. Evils lie behind such a house owner and his path of progress and rise is bedevilled by thorny problems.

Remedy

Dangle a mirror or an octagonal mirror on the back wall so that negative energy gets reflected in the mirror and wastes away.

A house at the corss roads

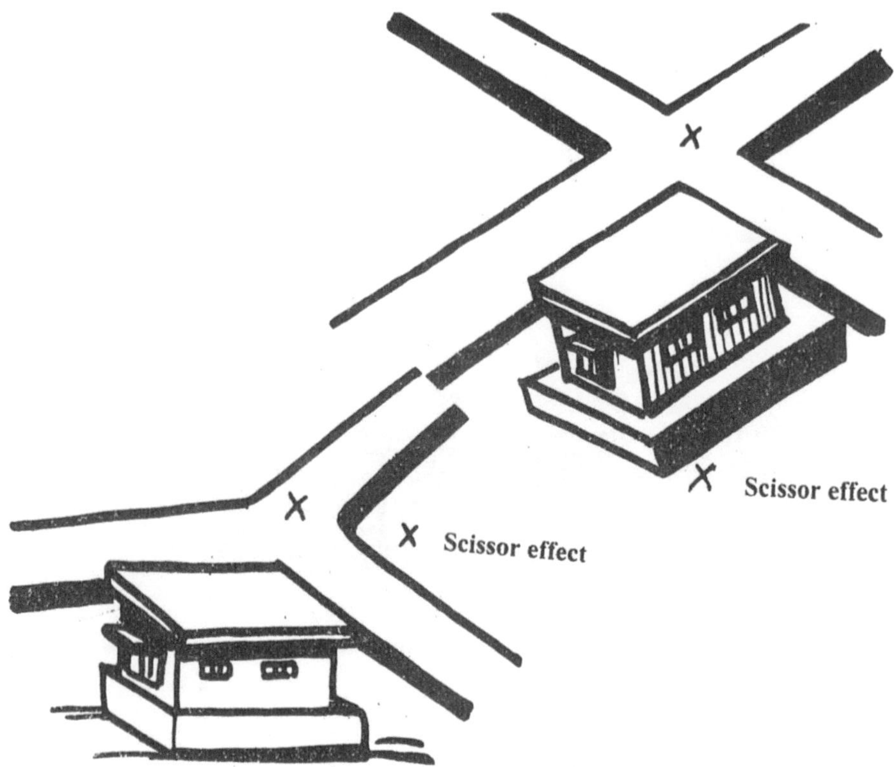

If a house is situated at the crossing of roads, (as shown in the above figures), it is not an auspicious sign because it indicates the house has been caught up between the scissors. According to Feng Shui it implies that negative energies are casting their ill effects on the house, due to which the dwellers in the house will meet with minor accidents. In foreign countries it is known as 'Scissor-effect house'.

Remedy

Plan and fix the door of the house in a corner in such a way that road should not look not be intruding into the house. Erect boundary wall, fencing or barrier outside the main gate and also fix an octagonal mirror on the wall that faces the main road.

A house built beneath a half-moon shaped circular bend or a culvert

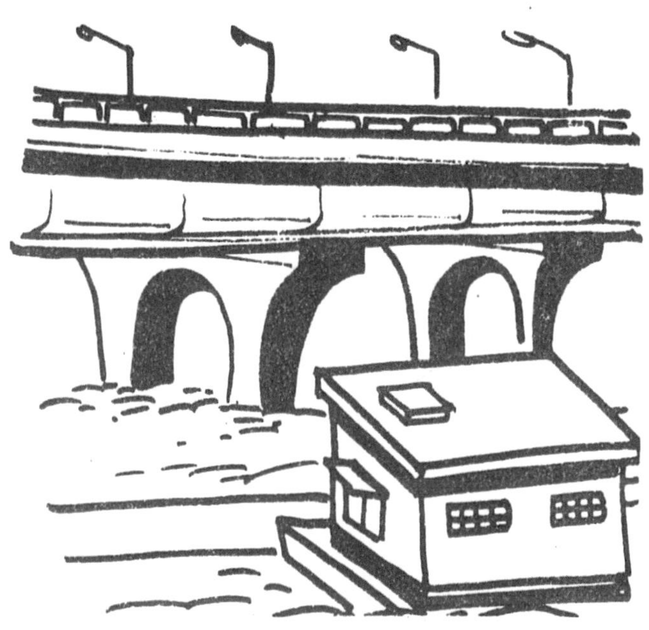

According to Feng Shui, it is an ominous sign if a house is built beneath semi circular turn, bridge, culvert or a railway crossing, a result of which the house-owner will remain a pauper, and continue to grapple with financial stringency and related problems, he will do such works that he himself will be caged in his own den.

Remedy

Fix a looking mirror of large size at the back side of the wall wherein images of railways crossing and culvert could reflect, so that negative energies can be kept away.

A house built in the vicinity of the busiest National Highway

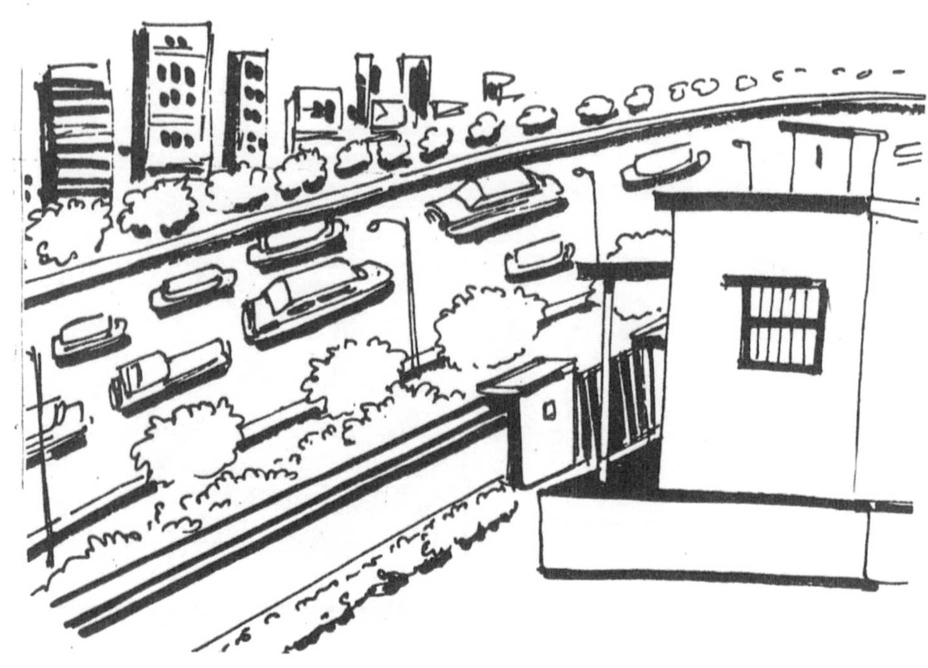

If your house is situated in the nearest vicinity of the busiest national highway and fast moving vehicles ply there on, it is not a suitable situation according to Feng Shui, due to which the house-owner will continue to reel under financial crunch and will not be able to save even a single penny.

Remedy

Do not construct the main door in the middle portion of the house, rather build the same in the corner, erect a boundary wall or barrier around the house so that positive energy can not escape and their negative energy can not let in. Dangle a mirror, an octagonal mirror on the walls which faces the national highway.

If a house is situated in front of an 'L'-Shaped Road

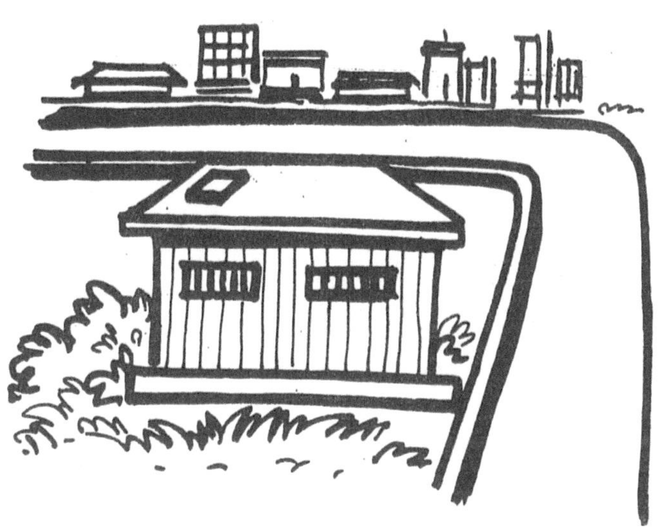

If any house is situated, (as shown is the above figure) in front of an L-shaped road, it is considered a bad location in Feng Shui. The owner of such a house will be manifested by such persons who will burden the house owner with their woes and personal problems.

Remedy

Dangle a high quality mirror or an octagonal mirror outside the house. Slightly raise plinth of the platform of the main gate.

If a house is surrounded by roads on all sides

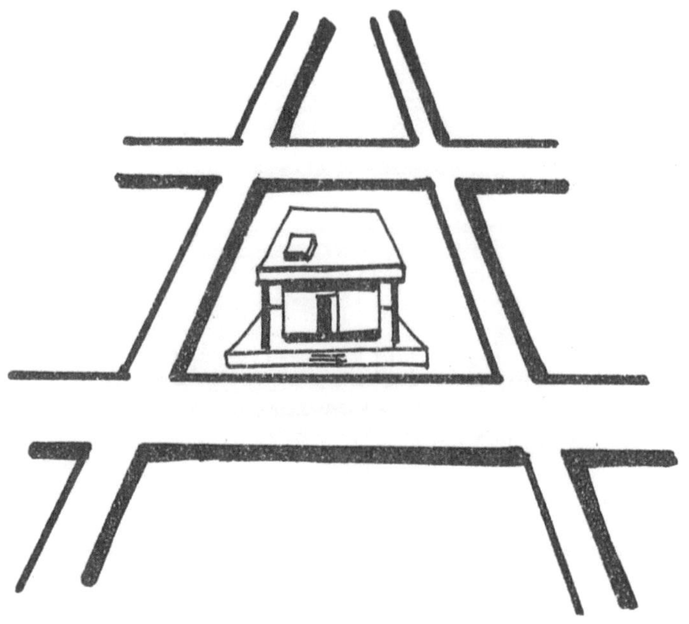

If a house is built at such a junction where it is surrounded by roads on all sides, then this it not an auspicious position according to Feng Shui and due to its impact entire life of the house owner will continue to be spent on useless matter and that he will not be able to make any saving.

Remedy

Raise the plinth of the house and its main gate is such a house should be after a height of 2-3 stairs.

When a house is built outside a roundabout

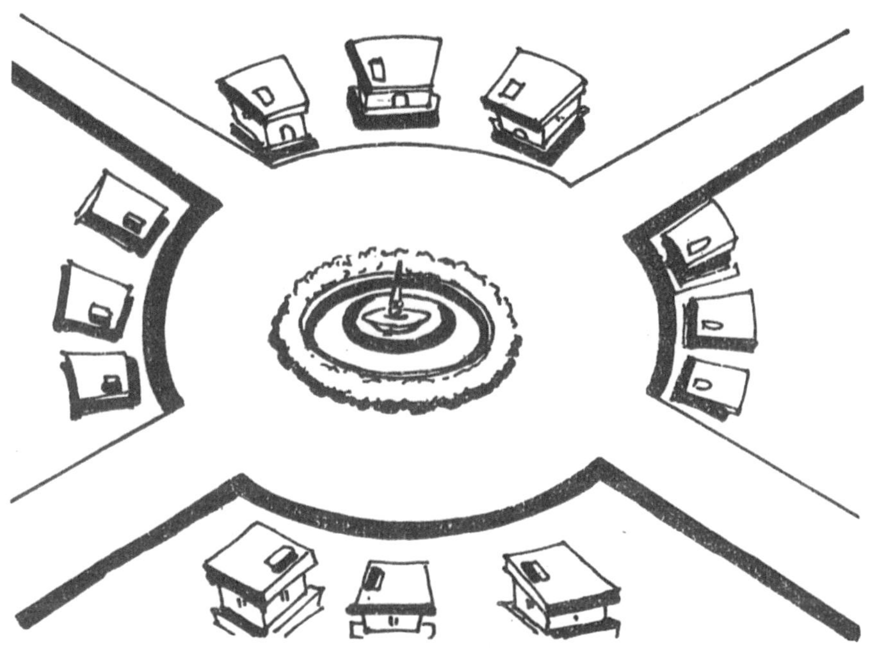

It is a good situation in Feng Shui if a house is built outside a round-about as it will enhance the house-owner's wealth, property and fame.

When corner of a house or bedroom is situated towards the road-side

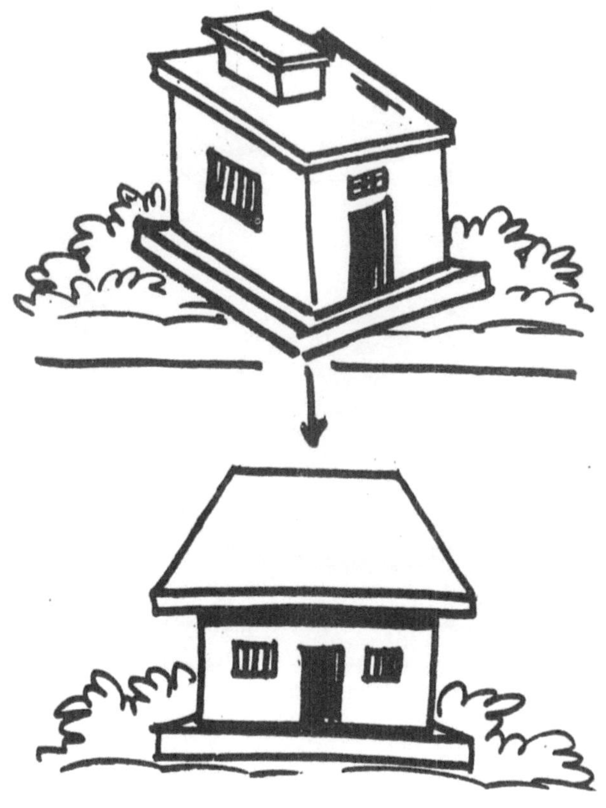

In Feng Shui it is not considered an auspicious sign, if corner or bedroom of a house falls towards the road (highway). The house owner in such a house will remain indisposed.

Remedy

Change the directional position of the bedroom or affix plastic blends on the door and windows. Feng Shui of the bedroom should be accorded special attention, because a person spends half of his life span in it; and it is the place where a person takes rest daily and acquires new strength and energy.

When a big building stands in front of a small house

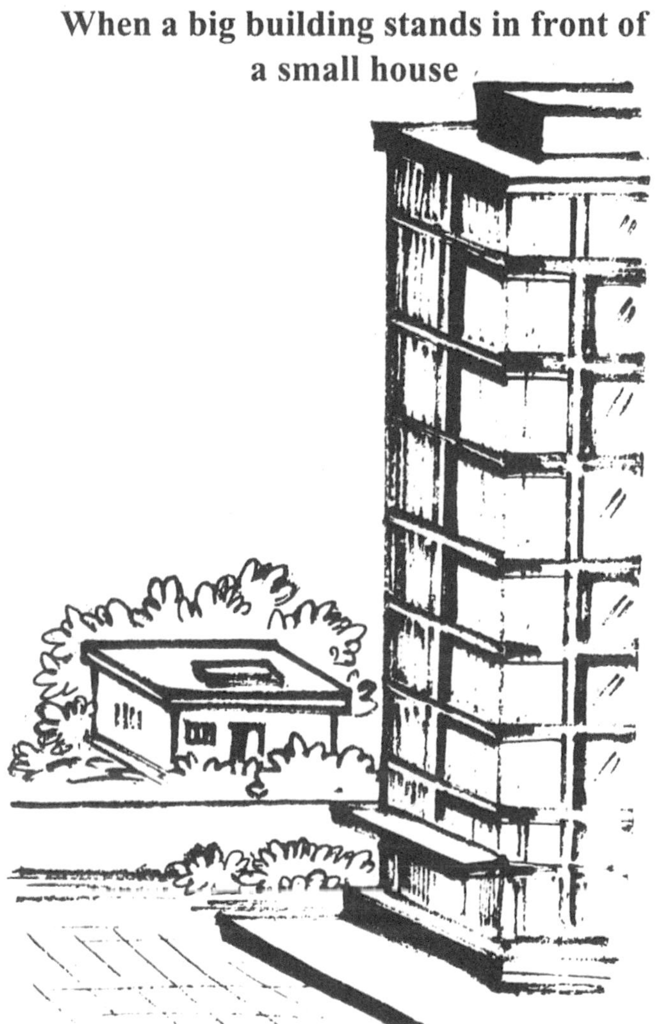

If a large-sized building is facing your smaller house or when construction work is in progress in the new building, such a situation is considered an impedimental factor to your residental house. In Feng Shui this situation is not considered auspicious. There will be theft or swindling on a large scale, and that too quite frequently.

Remedy

Do not keep your door opened. Put up a curtain over the main door and affix an octagonal mirror outside the main entrance gate.

If a burial ground is situated opposite a house

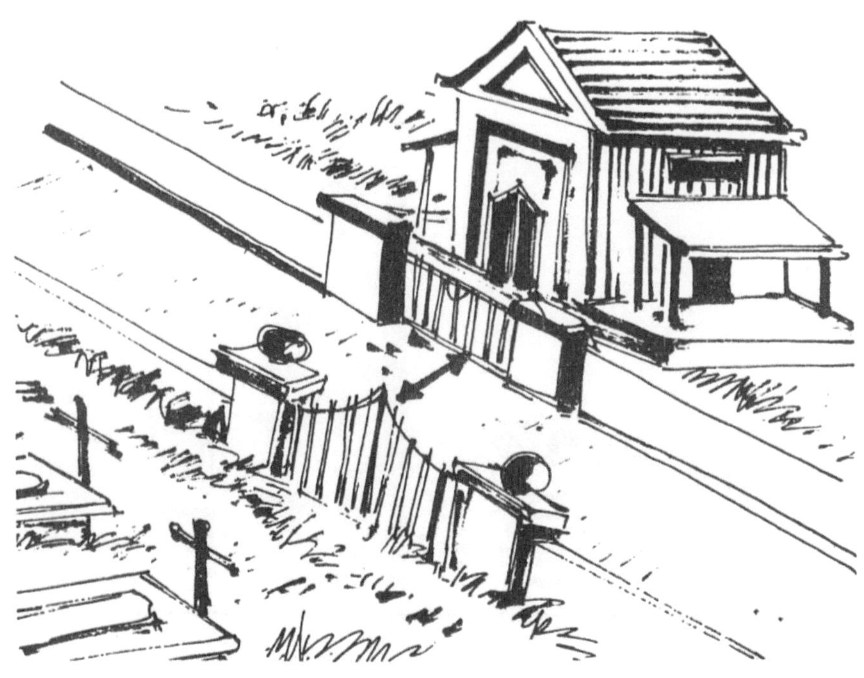

If a burial ground or ground where dead are burnt or it a hospital building exists in the front of the house, it is an ominous sign according of Feng Shui. Such a house will be an abode of illnesses, multiple problem will manifest there and the dwellers will not have a continuous and peaceful sleep.

Remedy

Keep a zero-watt bulb switched on always. If such a lamp keeps on lighting the place of worship, it will be still better.

If a church is situated opposite a house

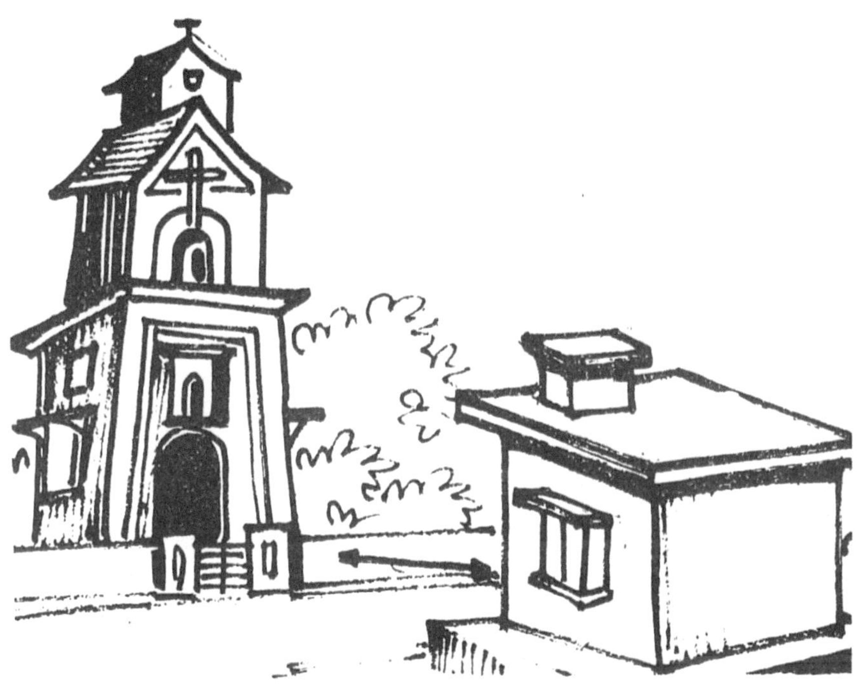

In Feng Shui science existence of a church opposite a residential house is an inauspicious sign; as such a situation keeps the house-owner agitated, angry and restive, and also renders the house a secluded place, because the number of inmates will gradually continue to windle.

Remedy

Fix an octagonal mirror outside the house so that the negative energy is dispelled or sent back after dashing against the mirror.

When an electric pole is situated opposite of a house

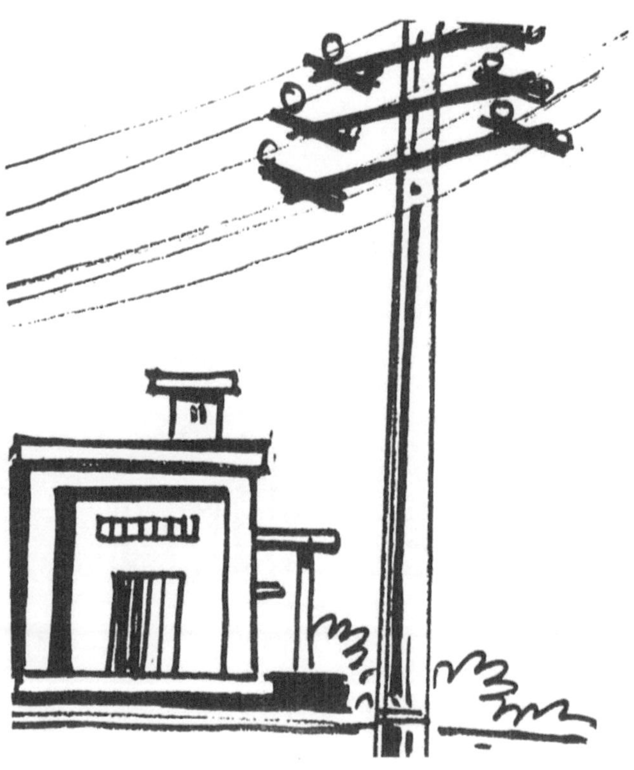

If an electric pole or a transformer exists opposite to a house, it is not an auspicious sign in Feng Shui parlance. The dwellers in such a house will always remain ill, there will be fears and court cases and the residents will suffer from fear psychosis of fire.

Remedy

Affix an octangonal mirror outside your house so that the negative energy is dispelled.

If a large gate or big pole exists in front of a house

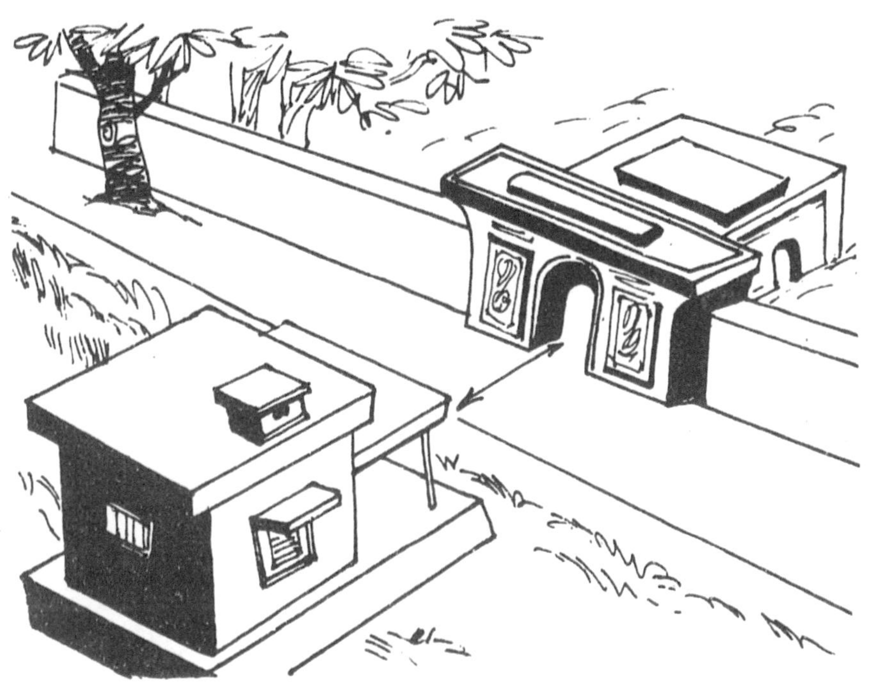

Existence of a big gate or pole in front of a house is not considered auspicious in Feng Shui, because residents of such a house will often fall ill, and their efforts will not yield expected results.

Remedy

Shift the main gate of your house to the corner so that it does not face the big pole or gate, or affix and octagonal mirror outside the house so that negative energy gets reflected to the original place from where it had originated.

If Shadow of a round dome of a house falls on a house

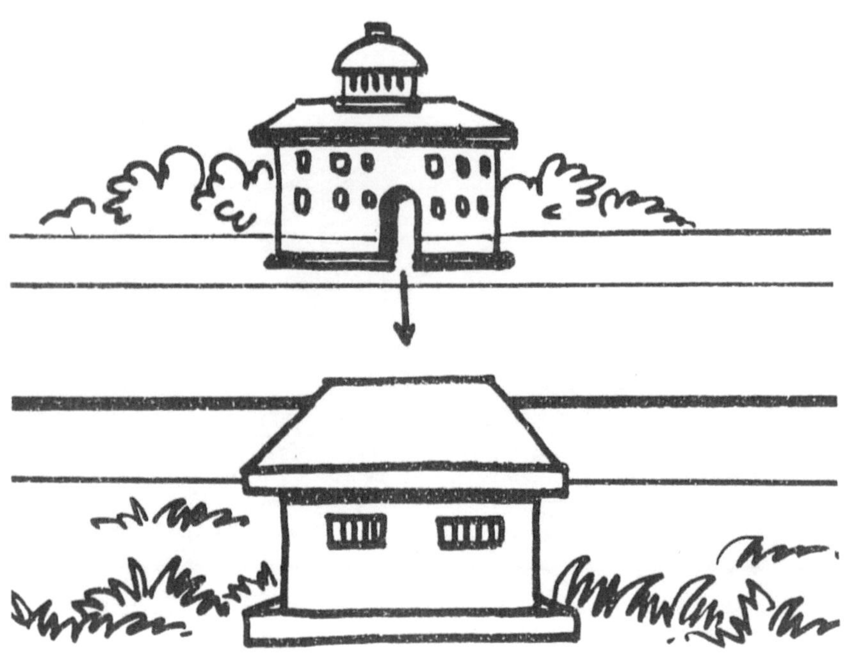

It is bad and harmful as per Feng Shui if shadow of a round-domed house falls on your house; bedroom or main gate. It is held that children, being in such a house, will be immoral and rascals and will fail to achieve their goals.

Remedy

It may be noted that harmful impact of a dome's shadow can not be cast upon the elderly persons but on the children only; hence the elderly persons have their bedroom in that direction, but the bedroom of children should be shifted to some others place where shadow of the domed house does not fall. Also affix and octagonal mirror on the main entrance gate.

Shadow of a triangle-shaped house falling on another house or its main door

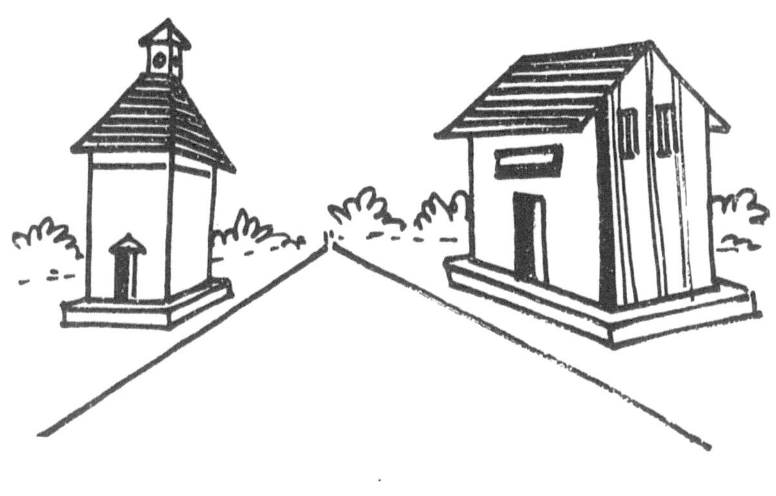

It is an ominous sign according to Feng Shui if shadow of triangular (triangle shaped) house falls on the main gate of bed room of your house. The persons sleeping in such a bedroom will continue to reel under fear of accidents.

Remedy

Use a curtain or plastic blades on the window of the bedroom and affix and octagonal mirror on the main gate.

Distance or Gap between two houses

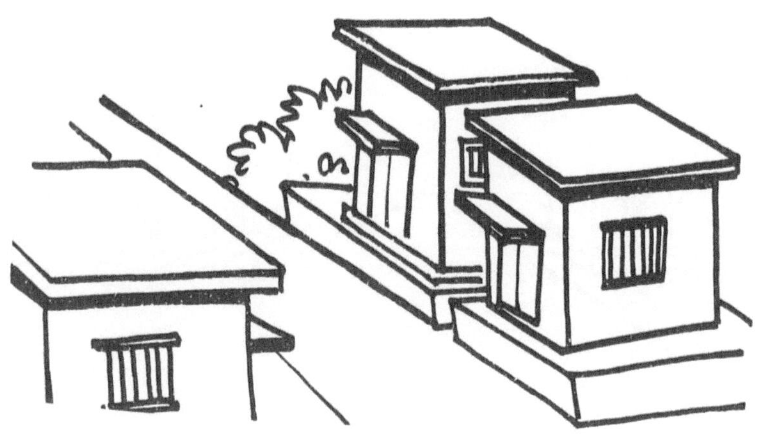

If houses are situated opposite to a house and gap between the houses is unequal, it is not considered a good sign in Feng Shui, as the residents in such a house will reel under fear of accidents and their health will also be a cause of concern.

Remedy

In order to discount ill effect of odd gaps and distances and also to stop entry of negative energy in the house, raise plinth level of the door at least by 2"— it will serve as a barrier and also stop entry of negative energy into the house.

22
Visiting Cards in accordance with Feng Shui

According to Feng Shui if you get visiting cards printed, their use will add to your name and fame and you will also have an effective public relations. In order to make an effective and lively visiting card, you should follow certain guidelines provided by astrology and Vaastu Shastra so that your contacts multiply.

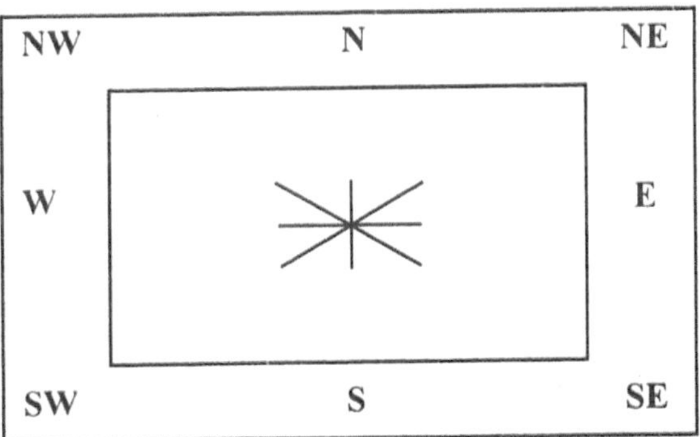

Let us first of all dwell upon size of a visiting card. According to Vaastu Shastra the size of the visiting card should be a right-angle one as a card having odd and uneven angles, can make any person tense, or disputable and can also snap away even the contacts. Hence a right-angled visiting card is always considered auspicious and most appropriate.

The second point pertains to knowledge about right directions. For instance, telephone numbers, fax numbers, mobile number and other contact numbers should be mentioned in the north-west corner and north central place you can mention your name in the central part, because this is a centre-point (Bramha-Sthaan) or due to want of proper space, you can also utilise lower part of south-west or western-central part also for the same purpose. You can also mention here name and address of your business.

If you do, as suggested, it will be auspicious and gainful. You can pick any type of card as per your preferred choice, or you can use a vertical card. Never give, torn punctured, dirty or distorted visiting card to anyone, as a mutilated and fragmented card will convert your success into failure.

Specimen of Visiting Cards.

For a best and flawless visiting card it is necessary that the centre-point of the card is kept written. In the north-east corner you can

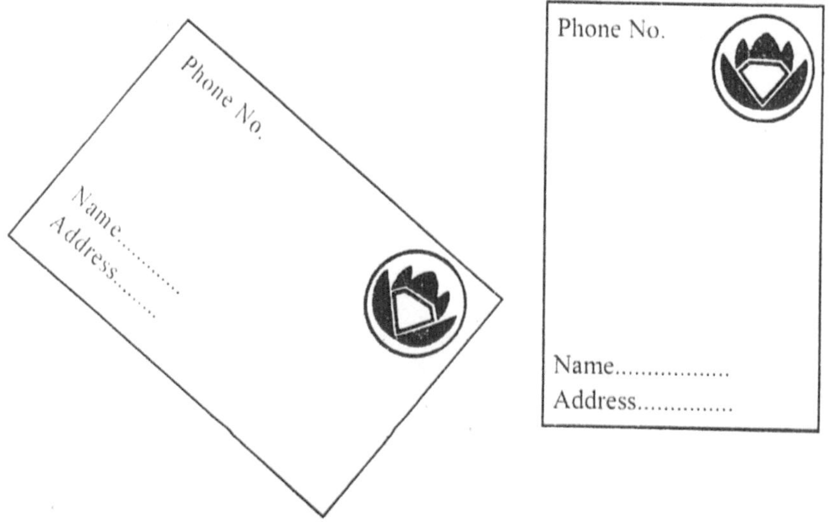

mention your trade mark, monogram in a vertical card or any other auspicious sign may be diagrammed. For instance you can use

'Swastik' sign, Ganpati's image, Sun or Mars etc. Colour in a visiting card should be in accordance with astrology. Ascertain from your horoscope which star is favourable or unfavourable. If you wish to use more than one colour, then you should use only depend on numerology where from you do not have your horoscope, you can depend on numerology where from you can ascertain your birth number, ruling number and the number of your name, lords of stars and suitable colours also.

Remember, an attractive card, if made according to relevant facts and rules of astrology or astronomy will service as an angle and helps to establish the contact with others.

❑❑❑

23

If Feng Shui is used properly, a maid servant will stage a comeback, who had deserted earlier

I have a foreign friend who has firm belief in Feng Shui, and occasionally he seeks my advise on certain matters in connection with Feng Shui. He and his wife are in an advanced age and they are a small family.

Their problem is, never a maid servant worked for them more than 6 months, even as they paid her a good salary.

They asked me whether there was any method in Feng Shui by which the maid servant, who had left the house, could come back? Their trusted maid servant had taken five hundred rupees on loan, but had not yet returned to work.

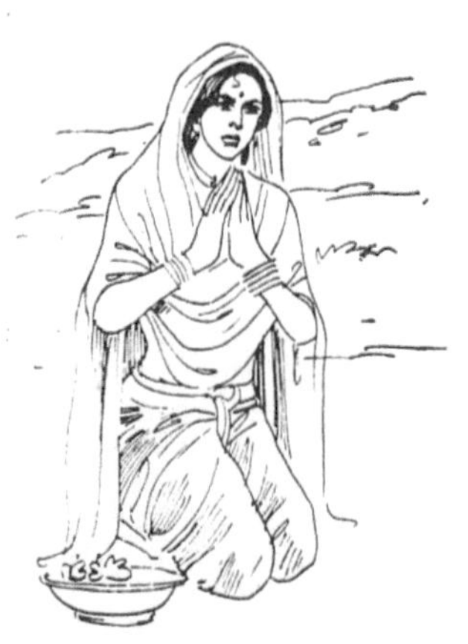

I examined their house with the help of a compass and found 3-4 electronic clocks and watchless laying idly in the corner of the house. These clocks were given to them by their friends.

The clocks were abandoned at a place in the house, which was not in use. All the clocks were new and lying unused in a corner and without battery.

According to Feng Shui directions, do not keep any clock or watch without battery in the house, otherwise servants and helping friends will discard you. I put cells in all the watches and made them functional. Next day a miracle happened. The maid servant returned and prayed to be forgiven for her wrong action. Thereafter she resumed her duties.

According to Feng Shui not only a big clock but even any other article, which is not in use, should never be kept in any house. Either mend the unused article or throw it away. But do not develop the habit of amassing useless articles in the house.

❑❑❑

24

Can Feng-Shui prove useful in ending feuds between a Daughter-in-law and Mother-in-law

There is hardly any place in the world where Daughter-in-law and Mother-in-law do not quarrel. I have studied the problem. I think the problem starts from the kitchen. In a kitchen of house, where a water tank is placed above the earth, such feuds occur rather commonly.

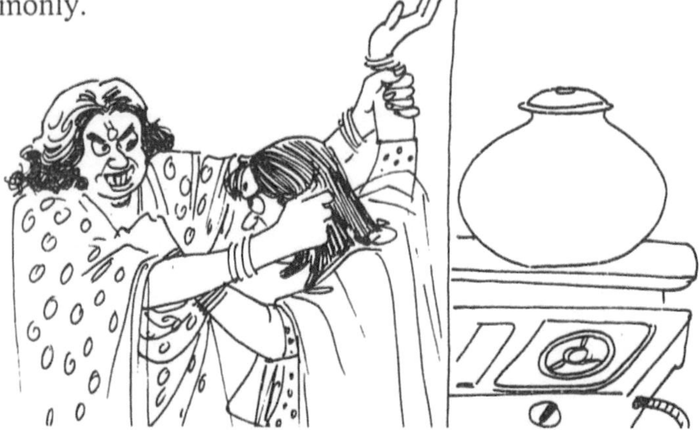

Once I went to Ahemdabad to visit a client. There the feud between the daughter-in-law and the mother-in-law was a regular feature in the family. Excuses and pretexts were picked up to start a quarrel. Even the husband was upset due to fighting between the two. All members also were affected due to the ongoing feud.

I examined to their kitchen where I noticed a water-tank above the gas-stove. I immediately understood root cause of the situation. Water and fire are opposite elements. Hence, the daily feuds were natural outcome. I used the compass and noticed that stove was in the south-east corner, but position of the water-tank was totally opposite to that. Both the said defects existed in their kitchen. Then I got the water-tank removed and shifted it to the north-east corner. A minor modification such as this can result in an end to mutual feud between the daughter-in-law and mother-in-law.

Though I also noticed that the mother-in-law was to be blamed and it was she who has poisoned the son and grand children against the daughter-in-law.

In 1996, I went to Jamnagar where a feud between the daughter-in-law and mother-in-law had gone to its worst, so much so that the family had almost decided to turn the daughter-in-law out of the home. The feuds even resulted in physical scuffles. The situation was tense and unmanageable due to ongoing squabbling, wherein entire blame was heaped on the daughter-in-law. Her mother-in-law, in fact, was so much upset that she even thought of committing suicide. I then took their daughter-in-law into confidence and talked to her in private where no one else was present. She related her woes and other problems. She never believed in feuds, but whenever she was angry she lost her cool and temper which she was unable to control. She also said that the quarrel always starts early in the morning before the time of tea, but situation remains normal from 10 a.m., to night. But, after taking the morning tea every member behaves normally. She also disclosed when she gets up there is heaviness in her head, she gets tense and wants to pick up quarrel with all and one. When she reprimanded and thrashed her children, they started crying and it was enough of a pretext for start the quarrel between her husband and mother-in-law.

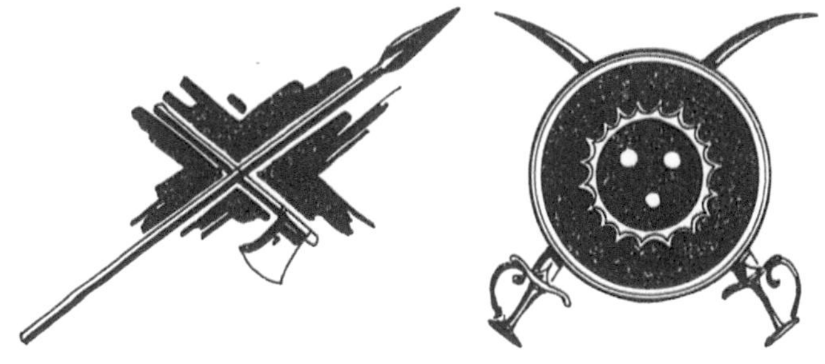

So, I came to the conclusion that cause of feud is not the kitchen but something else. I visited their bedroom and found a pairs of cross-swords (shown in the following figure) hanging on the wall.

In addition, there was a scenery from Mahabharat epic where it was shown that poor Abhimanayu was surrounded by mighty warriors and he was unable to defend himself—all these factors had poisoned the atmosphere in this family. Further, since the children, husband and wife slept in the same bed-room, their behaviour became rash and quarrelsome. It may be noted that atmosphere in the bedroom is the causative factor in triggering quarrels.

In the above situation everybody was bound to be adversely impacted. Then, after studying the situation and the ground realities I got impeding factors removed from the bedroom. If cross swords are found in any bedroom it will definitely result in feuds. I got all the anomalies removed in accordance with directions of Vaastu principles. Now the said family is living in peace, prosperity, tranquillity and amity.

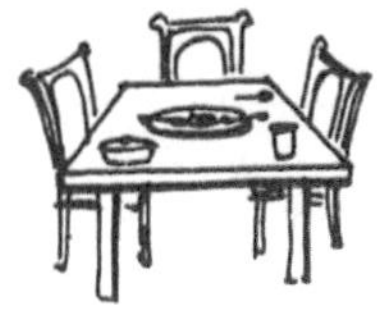

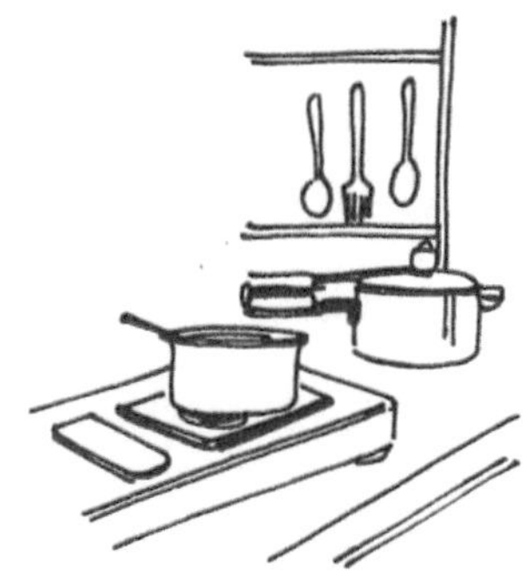

Not only this but it also matters a lot as to which type of furniture is kept in the kitchen and above all, their colours, because it also casts impact, good or bad, on the persons living in a house apart from affecting the general atmosphere in the family.

In 1998, I visited the house Chandrakant Bhai, a client's house. His family had 24 members which included sons, daughters,

daughters-in-law, son-in-law and grand children but they were unabale to get along, and there were ongoing feuds among the members. The cause of trouble was a new furniture in a new kitchen. I went to kitchen where there was an excellent combination of red and blue sunmica. Red colour denotes fire while the blue colour represents water, and there is an inherent and natural animosity between the colours. So, I advised them to modify the furniture in the kitchen according to Vaastru rules which he did as directed. I asked him to replace blue coloured sunmica with a yellow coloured one. Yellow is the representative colour of earth, and red, and yellow (fire and earth) colours are the naturally friendly colours. Such a minor change restored peace and mutual amity in the family.

Following points may be taken note of

❑ ***Your oven or toaster should never be kept over your refrigerator.***

❑ ***Do not keep water jugs, tea cup or fruit juice near your telephone instrument.***

❑ ***Whenever you have to use any colour, your selection of colours should be in accordance with advice and guidance of a Vaastu expert.***

❑❑❑

25
Can Feng-Shui help your daughter to get a suitable handsome husband?

I have undertaken thousands of visit in connection with Vaastu shashtra, Feng Shui and astrology. A common problem in most of the houses is that it is not easy to find a suitable match for their daughters. The same the problem about finding a suitable brides too.

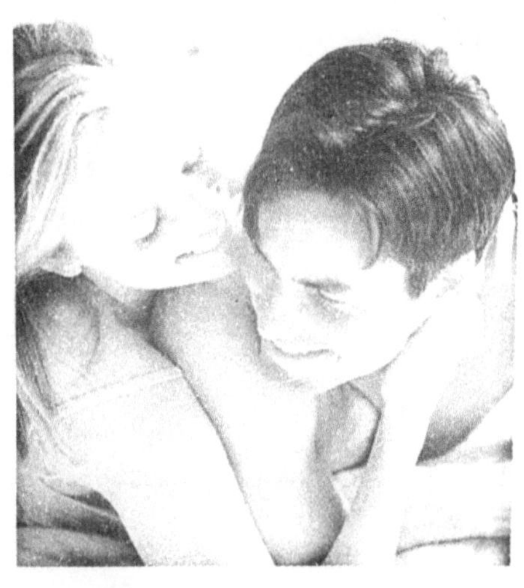

In respectable and affluent families even good looking educated and well employed boys reach the age of 35-40 yet unable to find a suitable match. The story is no different in the case of the girls. It is a tedious problem which persons like me have to face daily. Today's time is of fast-food culture, people have neither time nor patience, they have no belief in rituals and meditation. They want quick results.

However, they are not averse to direction. Once TV anchor inquired, during the course of an interview, whether there was any specific area in a house where a virgin (girl) should live so that she gets quickly married. I replied that it should be the north-west, the guests come and leave quickly. So, if a virgin girl's bed-room is made in the north-west direction and she lives therein, then she is most likely to get married soon. In Feng Shui, there are about 10-15 suggestions in this regard though all are not precise even then their important and utility can not be questioned and suspected.

For the benefit, of the readers I mention hereunder some of most effective and tried remedies which, if followed, will hopefully yield the desired results.

Some highly important formulae:

1. Do not ever keep trees, plants or flower-pots in the bedroom. According to Feng Shui, flowers, plants and branches belong to wood element and enhance Yang energy in the bedroom, hence excessive Yang energy an early marriage. It has also been mentioned in Feng-Shui that flowers of deep red and yellow colours should never kept in such a room where bachelor and virgins reside. These are ominous also. The Chinese never present bouquetes of red flowers to the patients. They present bunches having light yellow and white flowers, as they ensure quick recovery from illness.

2. According to Feng Shui never keep any TV or paper, pertaining to your profession, because such things create obstacles during happy moments of love-affairs.

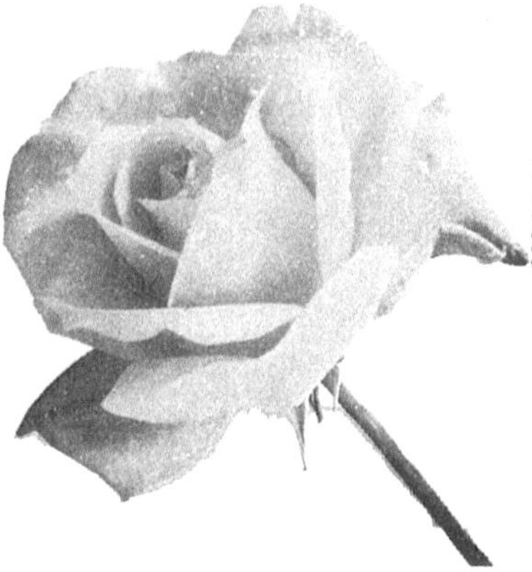

3. Rose considered as a symbol of love. But never present a thorny rose to your lover because, according to Feng Shui, thorn is an obstacle to love-affairs. Hence if a thorny rose is presented to a lover, it is like inviting one's misfortune. So, instead of presenting dark red coloured rose to a lover, present a throneless rose of light pink, orange or light yellow colour or a bunch of sunflower— it will enhance affection, romance and attraction. But all said and done, the Chinese consider a lotus as the beast presentation, as it promotes love-affairs. It is, of course, recommended in Feng Shui, as lotus flower is the most sacred medium to promote natural love and affection also.

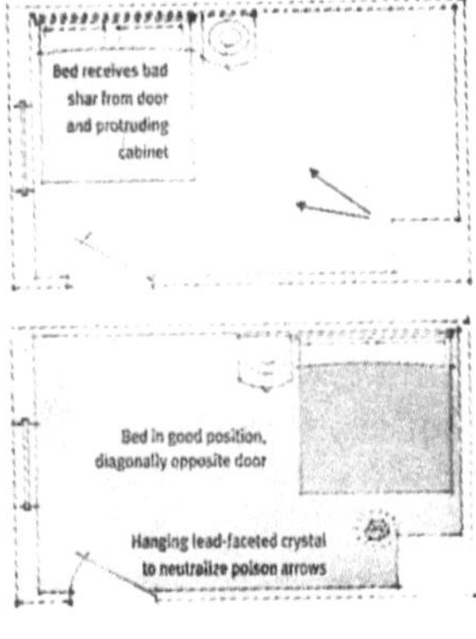

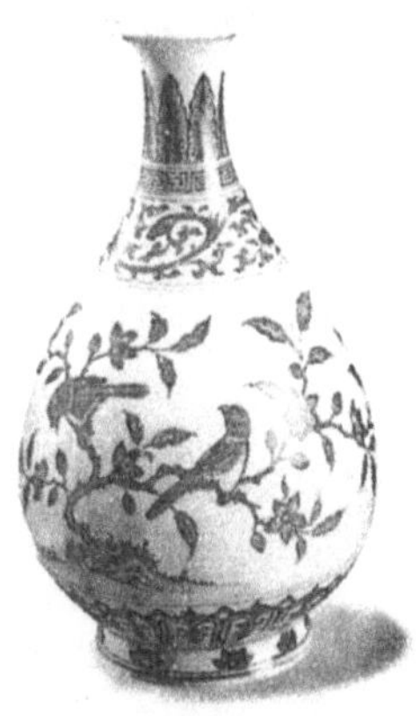

4. Special attention must be paid to the sleeping pattern of an unmarried person. Do not keep head and feet in front of a door. There should also be a beautiful crystal ball or an attractive pendant of an ear-ring in front of the head so as the attract a good partner, girl or a boy — it will also attract your fortune to your side. Or keep multi-coloured gems, costly stones, crystal or an attractive white ware or a piece of antique.

5. Dangle pictures of love-birds at the corner or wall of the bedroom. Keep also a pairs of love-birds at the place where marriage is (likely) to be performed. Also affix pictures of pairs of swan, duck, cuckoo, golden sparrows, pigeon, parrot, peacock etc as all these birds and their pictures help in finding out suitable and lucky partners for the unwed. In China and South-East Asia, people prefer to dangle picture of phoenix, which a divine and ancient birds, instead of the love-birds recommended in Indian Vaastu.

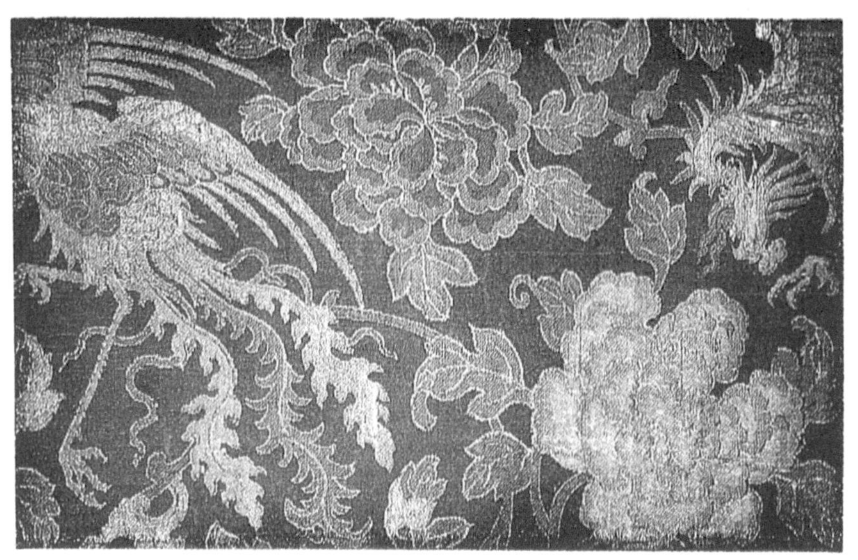

6. Keep light pink colour/paint of the walls and curtains.
7. If you are already betrothed or likely to be betrothed soon, and have also selected your partner according to your choice, then affix the following picture (depicting love-knot) in

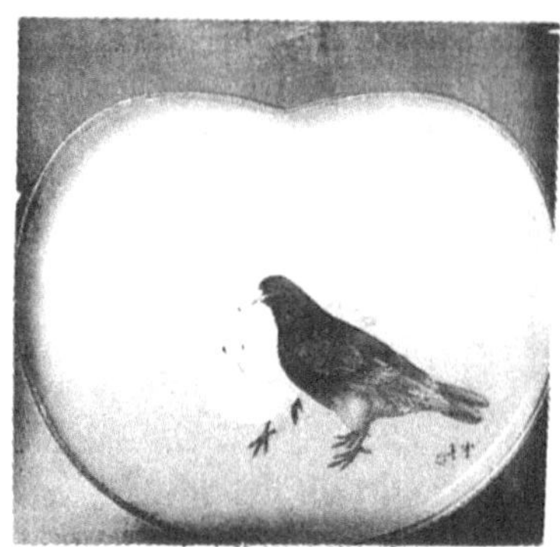

your bed-room—it will lead your love-affair to finality an after marriage you will lead a happy and successful marital life.

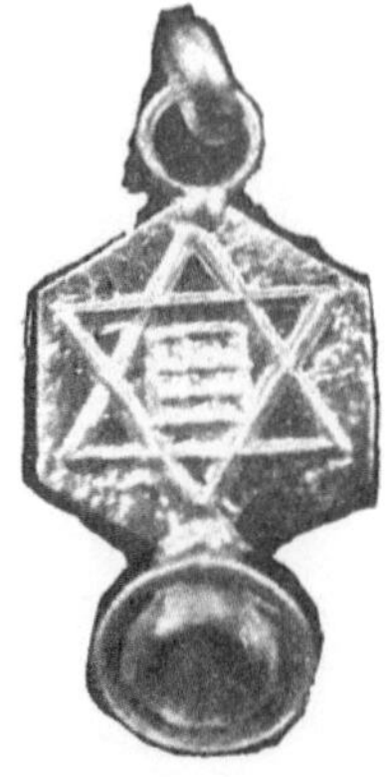

8. In addition to the most effective method is a diamond or Zircon-studies 'Shukra Yantra'* around your neck in the name of your fiance/fiancee. If a desirous person keeps fast on 28 Fridays, he will get his/her desired partner within three days, 45 days or three months. If you still want quicker results, the Hindus should ignite a deepak (an earthern lamp using cow-milk-made butter/ghee) in the temple of goddess on every Friday, the Muslims should ignite 9 earthens lamps (Chirag) in a mosque every Friday) using mustard oil, and the Christians should light 9 candles on every Sunday in a Church, the Hindus can also float two earthen lamp in the flowing water.

❑❑

* **Our readers can contact the author directly to obtain a 'Shukra Yantra' or get further information about Feng Shui. They may laso read the book, entitled 'Vaastu Jigyaasaayen Aur Samaadhaan' published by *'DIAMOND POCKET BOOK.'***

Terminology of Feng Shui

A

1. An Lu:-It denotes south-west direction which ensures excellent health, leisure, comforts prosperity, peace etc, which are necessary ingredients for a family's happiness.
2. Arrowed killing Chi:- These are two or more straight lines, within which 'Chi' (The mystical power) flows.
3. Azyre dragon:- According of Chinese belief, it is an auspicious sign of dragon which denotes safety and protection hence it is used in all the treaties, this symbol is also always affixed on the left side of the Chinese temple.

B

1. Bagua:- It is an amulet (Talisman or a mystical diagram) which consists of eight Trigrams, as it denotes eight powers.
2. Bing:- It is one of the 10 "Stems". It implies "Root of Progress".
3. Buddhism:- A religion propounded by Lord Buddha. Though it originated in India but spread and popularised more in China, Singapore, Hongkong, Bangkok and (other Asian countries).
4. Black Hat Sect:- It is a bigoted/fanatical organization, Tibetan Tantrik Buddhism .It fervently believes in Taoism, Confucians, ancient mass therapy, Loteine and Feng Shui and utilises these disciplines to treat medical cases on mass basis.

C

1. Chai:- A residential building.
2. Chakra:- An epicentre of energy or power.
3. Chang Yen:- Western direction whose winds impact happiness and good health.

4. Chen:- A rising Trigram whose associate elements are cold, north-east direction, wood and electricity.
5. Ch'i:- A mystical natural power.
6. Ch'i:- It is a constructive Trigram whose chief attributes are heat, fire, heaven and south direction.
7. Chin:- It represents Feng Shui's fourth elements, that is "wood".
8. Chin TS'a: Its attributive elements are friendliness and auspicious move.
9. Chin-Yen:- North direction, new relations.
10. Chinese Animal Year:- In China; every Chinese year represents an animal and the process repeats itself after every cycle of twelve years. Their serial is as follows- 1. Dragon 2. Snake 3. Horse 4. Goat 5. Monkey 6. Cow 7. Dog 8. Pig 9. Mouse 10. Bull or Ox 11. Tiger 12. Hare.
11. Chuch-Ming:- Completely harmful sign.
12. Chon:- It is one of the twelve branches which implies reproductivity and budding.
13. Chu-Shr:- This is a therapy, which is beyond the realm of science, logical conclusions, and the treatment is conducted by means of scintillating and wondrous methods.
14. Cosmic Breath:- It means good life-giving wind. (In Indian Parlance "Prana"). The Chinese believe that even the dead bodies buried in a house requires good (Prana-Vayu) cosmic breath (say oxygen). It is also called as "Supernatural Cosmic breath".
15. Command Position:- It means the best position for placing a bed or desk in a room but neither of these objects should be placed in front of the opening of the door.

D

1. Dharma:- In Feng Shui Dharma means "Buddha Dharma".
2. Di-ji-Jea:- The Chinese Feng Shui expert who foretells future after examining the land or place.
3. Di-Li:- Chinese Feng Shui.
4. Ding:- It is one of the ten 'stem' which means "Ripeness or Maturity".
5. Di-Zhi:- It pertains to twelve branches of Geology in respect of knowledge about land.
6. Double Hours:- The Chinese divided 12 hours into a span of two hours each, which is as follows:-

   Chou— 1 a.m. to 3.00 a.m., Yen 3.00 a.m. to 5.00 a.m.

E

1. Enrichments:- The term generally implies 'achievements' but for the Chinese it is a technical term that refers to a specific gadget that denotes eight perspectives. These are eight Trigrams constructed by means of this instruments and these separate Trigrams are called "Eight Encroachments".
2. Eight Trigrams:- These were originated in 2852 B.C. by Fu HSien which denote eight points in the compass.

F

1. Fa Chan:- The eastern direction.
2. Fan Ch'i:- Negative Energy.
3. Fang:- Internal.
4. Feng:- Wind element.
5. Feng Husang:- A mythological bird of red hue who is the lord of southern direction. According to the Chinese belief it is one of the four divine and heavenly birds.
6. Feng Shui H Sien-Sheng:- A professional Feng Shui expert who explains Feng Shui.
7. Fu-Wei:- A condition for personal progress.

G

1. Geomancy:- Feng-Shui,
2. Geomancer:- Feng-Shui scholar.
3. Geng:-It is one of the ten stems. It means changes inclined towards completion.
4. Giog Hong Tian:- This is the title of a Chinese Temple which is situated at Heaven Road, Singapore.
5. Gua:- It is one of the Trigrams of eight angled Bagua emulet.
6. Guan Di:- Lord/Deity of war, a great warrior who ruled over three capdats and also enjoyed.
7. Guan Ying Tong:- A famous Chinese temple which is at Singapore's Bataugab Drive.

H

1. Hai:- It is one of the twelve branches which means change.
2. Hexagram:- It is a hexagonal sign which forms two Trigrams, representing specific situations. There are 64 formations of Hexagram which have been explained in details in the

chapter titled 'I'-Ching.

3. Hong San Temple:- It is a Chinese Temple, situated in Mohd. Sultan Road, in Singapore.
4. H'Sun:- This is a Trigram which represents wind and its assisting faculties are extreme heat, wood element and south-west direction.
5. H Sen:- Heart.
6. H Suen:- It means all-around.
7. Huna Lo:- South-east direction (Agniya).
8. Huo:- Fire.
9. Hu-Lu:- A magical achievement of the Chinese by, the use of which evil spirits are contained.

I

1. I-Ching:- It is an ancient book on the Chinese culture and astrology, also called 'The Book of Change'. This book was written 3000 years ago; Wherein one gets a glimpse of Chinese ancient philosophy and the art of prediction. It is based on eight Trigrams out of which 64 Hexagrams are formed.

J

1. Jen Hsen:- Central point.
2. Ji:- It is one of the ten stems which means "Freedom".
3. Jea:- It is also one of the ten stems and means "Emblem or sign of progress".

K

1. Kabhallah:- It is the name of traditional Jewish umbrella or is the term used for spiritual or philosophical sittings or congregations.
2. K'an:- It is the name of dangerously Trigram which is assisted by western direction, spring season, metal element and the moon.
3. Kan-Yu-Jea:- An adept in Feng Shui art.
4. Ken:- Trigram of the mountain whose (assisting) attributes are cold, south-west direction and cold season.
5. Killing Ch'i:- It is an ominous energy or power that runs rapidly through straight lines.
6. Kua Number:- According to Feng Shui, every person has a

Kua number, on the basis of which he can modify and change favourable or unfavourable directions. Kua number is determined according to dates of lunar year, but Kua numbers of man and win are different.

7. Kui:- It forebodes advent of spring season.
8. K'un:- It is a significant Trigram, related to winter. North direction, water element and constructive tendency.

L

1. Lao-Zi:- He was a religious leader and philosopher, who was contemporary of Confucius, and founded "Taoism" between 551- 497 B.C.. This is a religious sect where principle of universal fraternity has been propounded for the welfare of humanity.
2. Leon San See:- This is a famous Chinese temple, situated at Race Course Road, Singapore, which I visited during my tour of Singapore.
3. Li:- It is a Trigram which is related to spring, eastern direction, wood element and the Sun.
4. Ling:- It is an upraised arrow of natural power "Chi" or a symbol of uprising soul prior to death.
5. Liu:- Tree, garden, stem of a tree.
6. Lo pan:- A magic square, measuring 3x3 (=9).
7. Lo Shu:- Wherein numerical numbers, from 1 to 9, are written in such a way that the total will come to 15, when added and counted from any side. In India we call it "Panariya Yantra".
8. L ong:- It means 'Dragon' which is indicative of nature's positive energy. It is Chinese ancient custom to keep picture of idol of dragon at auspicious site.
9. Loshu Grid:- Lakshami yantra, Panaruya.
10. Lou pan: It is a particular type of compass which indicates specifice details of astrological signs, as they appear in Feng Shui.
11. Lui-Sha:- Six numerous directions.
12. Lung mei:- Vein of Dragon through which the positive energy, "Chi", passes.

M

1. Mandala:- A circle- it is an instrument which is used by the Vaastu experts to hypnotise people, even while sitting at home.
2. Mantra:- It is a sacred recitation of pious words. If an aspirant repeatedly Chants a mantra, he will attain a special power.
3. Meo:- It is one of the twelve branches which means perfection.
4. Meridian:- It is a flow within which natural energy flows.
5. Mu:- It denotes "Wood" element which occupies second place amongst the fire elements.
6. Mudra:- Various sacred formations of hands, through which energy can be transferred.

N

1. Nien-Yen:- A direction that enhances "Romaa".

O, P

1. Pakua or Pa'Kwa:- This an octangonal instrument which contains eight Trigrams, and each Trigram has inherent mystical connotations. Positive energy in the house can be improvised with the help of this instrument.

Q

1. Qi:- It is power of nature's inhaling and exhaling process which constitutes this universe, including the mountains. It also imparts spiritual power to a person. It is also called "Chi".

R

1. Red Envelope:- According to Feng Shui "Red envelop" is a Chinese traditional method of treatment. A Feng Shui expert hands over this envelop to a family member who later takes it to 'The Yun Lin Temple' or dedicates it to his deity, in the temple at his home. So that the deity is able to remove Vaastu related defects. This author himself personally witnessed this type of treatment in the temples in Hongkong.
2. Ren:- It is one of the ten stems which means "Climax of the Festival".
3. Ru-Shr:- This is a type of therapy which is totally opposed to the logical and scientific therapy.

S

1. Seferoth:- It is tree of life-a cabbalistic symbol.
2. Sha:- A negative energy, barren earth/dust.
3. Sha Ch'i:- A negative energy that flows from the Western direction.
4. Shan:- A mountain.
5. Shan Shui:- Mountain and water. It is a specific Chinese picture in which scenes of mountain and water are painted.
6. Shao Yang:- East or weak Yang energy force.
7. Shad Yen:- West or weak yen energy / force.
8. Shao Qi:- Negative energy.
9. Shau:- It is one of the twelve branches which means "Origin from maturity".
10. Shen Ch'i.:- It implies a favourable direction or positive rays emanating from the eastern direction.
11. Shui:- Water element which has fifth and last position amongst the five elements.
12. Si:- It is one of the twelve branches which implies 'Dragon from perfection/maturity'.
13. Six TrueWorld:- It means 'Six true words' which the Feng Shui experts employ to remove defects in a house.
14. Song of Geomancy:- This book was written (in 400 B.C.) in twelve parts by Kuo-P'u which was also known as 'Book of Burial'.
15. Stupa:- This is sacred ladder which represents and consists of five elements, five power and five steps.
16. Sying:- It means visualising the science atmosphere and objects which we can perceive with our naked eyes with the aid of Feng Shui.
17. Syong-Huang:- It is an ominous power, which is used in Feng Shui for treatment. This power resembles red colour of Tu-Sha.

T

1. Tai Ch'i:- Ultimate supernatural power.
2. T'ai Ch'i Chuan:- Chinese art of numerology.
3. Tai Ji:- Great Power.
4. T'ai Yang:- Sun or southern direction of great Yang.

5. T'ai Yui:- Moon or northern direction of a great day.
6. Tao:- This is the name of a particular religion, sect or community and philosophy.
7. Taoism:- Tao Religion.
8. Ten Stens:- Its synonymous name is "Tean Gan" which is a technical term which was used from 1766 B.C. in place of Taoism. Yen objects relating to heaven are known as "Ten Stars".
9. Thain Hock Kong:- This is a famous Chinese temple (which the author himself visited in 1981) is situated at Tallock Aiyar Street in Singapore.
10. T'ien Ch'ai:- It means north-east direction ('Ishaan') which relates to family and children.
11. Tong Shu"- This is an astrological calendar of the Chinese which has been in vogue since 2200 B.C., which includes details regarding Chinese festivals, dates for marriage, dates for worshipping the ancestors (dead), Chinese traditional celebrations, and forecasts about the seasons.
12. Tien Yi:- The direction that enhance health.
13. Trigram:- This Diagram consists of three transverse lines whose position varies in each Trigram-the upper line stands for heaven, the middle line denotes humanity and the lowest line denotes earth element.
14. T' Sang Ch'i:- Mysterious waves emitting from the northern direction.
15. T' Sang Feng:- It is a mysterious cold wind which blows from within a hole and causes illness to people.
16. T.T.B:- It is Tibetan Tantrik based on emulates Buddhism which is taken to 'Black Hat Sect' with have faith in treating various ailments by means of tantra, magic and Feng Shui.
17. T'u:- Earth element.
18. Twelve Branches:- In Chinese it is called as "Di Zhi". In 1766 B.C. twelve branches of knowledge, pertaining to earth, came into existence.

U

V

W

1. Walk Hai Cheng Beo:- This is a famous Chinese temple, situated at Philips Street, Singapore, which is like an institute where Feng Shui is studied. The author visited this temple, in 1986, for the purpose of study, during his visit to Singapore.
2. Wang TS'al:- Western direction which yields fame and prosperity.
3. Wei:- It is one of twelve branches of study that pretents to knowledge about the earth, which implies "identification of a perfect target".
4. Wen:- Eastern direction's lord, that is green dragon, which according to ancient Chinese beliefs, is one of the four divine animals.
5. White Tiger:- According to ancient Chinese beliefs white Tiger imparts high class auspiciousness, hence it is a sign of auspicious due to this beneficial characteristic of the white Tiger, its picture is put on the buildings. It is also the lord of western direction.
6. Wu:- White Tiger is the lord of the Western direction, as per Chinese ancient beliefs, and is one of the divine animals or it is also considered as one of the "Ten Stans" which means. "Perfect or Complete".
7. Wu H Sing:- It denotes progress five elements viz, wood, fire, earth, metal and water.
8. Wu Xing:- "Wu" means "Five" and "Xing" means "Five" mobile elements so this entire term means "Five mobile elements" which serially are described in this order- 1. Wood 2. Fire 3. Air 4. Earth 5. Water.

X

1. Xiang- Decoration of burial place, as per directions given in Feng Shui.
2. Xing:- To proceed, walk and move.
3. Xen:- It is one of the ten stems which means return to the previous position.
4. Xue:- It is sort of hole but, according to Feng Shui, this hole points out to foundation of a grave.

Y

1. Yang:- Of the two different power bestowed by nature, it is

a positive energy, which helps to constitute this universe. It is energy and its element is male. It remains aligned to Yeng energy.

2. Yang Ch'i:- A positive energy that animals from the southern direction.
3. Yi:- It is one of the ten stems which means "Expansion or distention of progress".
4. Yi Ting:- It is a book that contains principles pertaining to the ever changing world. This is an ancient book, authored by Chinese superior, Fu Zi where in an attempt has been made to visualise eternal changes that occur in human life, by way of 64 pictorial figures.
5. Yin:- This helps towards formation of entire universe but it is a negative force. Its element is female and lives in darkness. The energy remains aligned to "Yang" energy.
6. You:- It is one of the twelve branches which means "Accomplishment".
7. Yuan Wu:- It means tortoise, the lord of the northern direction. According to the Chinese beliefs, tortoise is one of the four divine animals of the heaven.

Z

1. Zhui Zi:- This is the name of a renewed Chinese scholar and theologist who had faith in the Tao sect and was quite popular in 300 B.C.
2. Zha Yuan Zhang:- He was the first emperor of the Yang dynasty.
3. Zi:- It is one of the twelve branches which means 'A new bud of a plant'.

Gratitude

Till now I have written 126 books on topics Vaastu, Astrology, Yantra, Mantra, Tantra—— Karmakaand, Kalasarpayoga, Hindu beliefs in traditions, Feng Shui. I am fortunate that the vast majority of the readers have recognised my humble efforts, as I continue to receive letters, telephone calls, fax messages etc. from them, and to my best to set at rest-their inquisitiveness. Friends, admirers, scholars have approbated my contribution to Vaastu, Astrology, Hinduism and Feng Shui. I am particularly obliged to Shri Narender Kumar Ji, Managing Director of Diamond Pocket Books, who motivated me to write this book in Hindi. I am also obliged to Pt. Shiv Sharma Ji for translation of this book into English.

I am also obliged to the writers and scholars whose books have stood me in good stead. Hence I express my grateful thanks and sense of gratitude to all of them. I have used the following books as refrence books.

Bibliography

1. **Feng Shui for Business,** by Avlen Lipp.
2. **Feng Shui for the Home,** by Avlen Lipp.
3. **Feng Shui for the Pillars of Destiny,** by Raymond Lo.
4. **Feng Shui and Destiny for Marriage,** by Raymond Lo.
5. **Chinese Geomancy,** A layman's guide by Avlen Lipp.
6. **Chinese Number,** by Avlen Lipp.

Note: All the books, S.No. 1 to S.No. 6 have been published by Time Book International, Singapore,

7. **Feng Shui Today**— Jami Linn, Published by B. Jain Publishers, New Delhi.
8. **The Feng Shui Kit**—Man Ho Koak.
9. **Change For Life Feng Shui**—B.Jain Publishers.
10. **Feng Shui**—A Mine of Information—Richard Craze.
11. **Feng Shui The Chinese Art of Placement**—
12. **Feng Shui at Igileson**—Lillin too.
13. **The Complete Guide to Feng Shui**—Gill Hallay.
14. **Feng Shui Workbook**—Wu Xing.
15. **Interior Design with Feng Shui**—Rider.

In addition of the authors of above mentioned books, I am also grateful to newspapers, magazines, journals. I also thank those persons whose name I am unable to mention, and also those who, directly and indirectly, inspired me during my visit to foreign countries to write this book. I am confident that the discerning readers will certainly find this book informative and also that it will solve many of their doubts on Feng Shui. Hopefully, this book will prove a milestone.

❑❑❑

NEW PUBLICATIONS

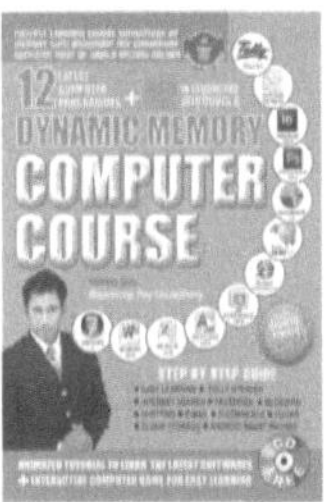

Biswaroop Roy Chowdhury
Dynamic Memory Computer Course **(Updated & Revised)**

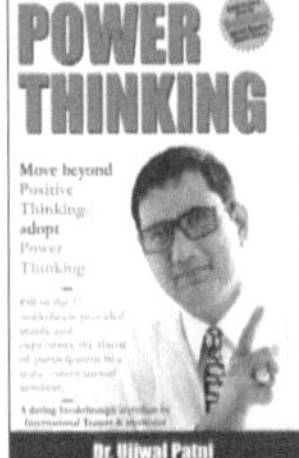

Dr. Ujjwal Patni
Power Thinking

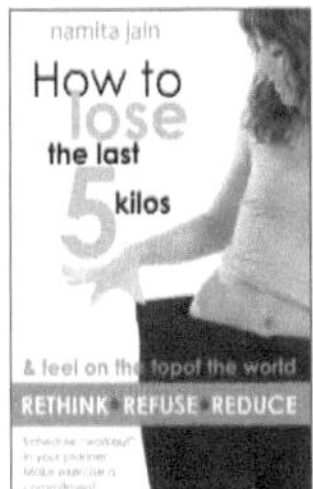

Namita Jain
How to Lose the last 5 Kilos

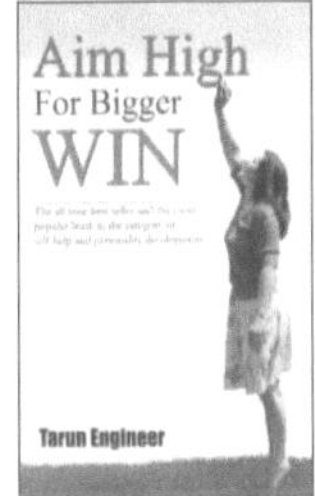

Tarun Engineer
Aim High For Bigger Win

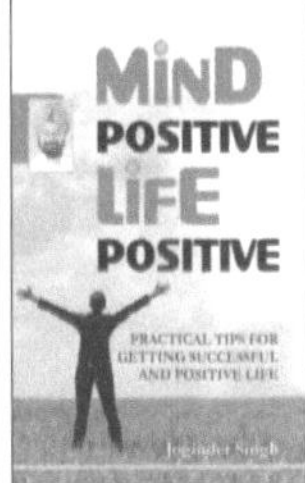

Joginder Singh
Mind Positive Life Positive

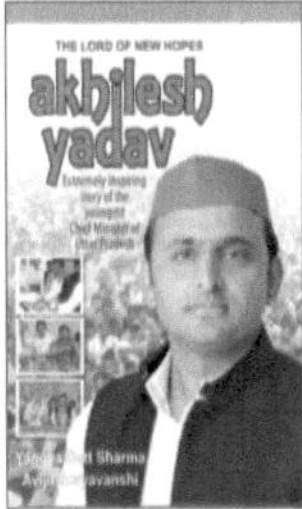

Yaggya Dutt Sharma
The Lord of New Hopes Akhilesh Yadav....

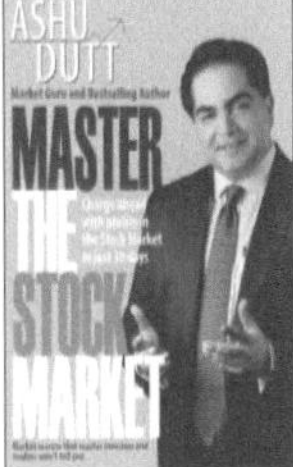

Ashu Dutt
Master the Stock Market

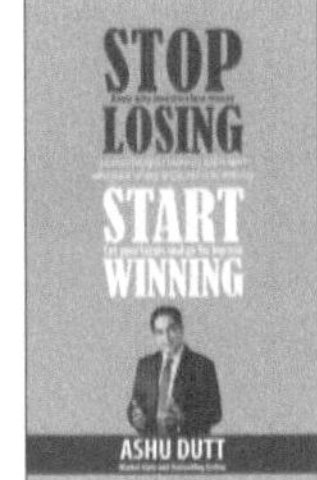

Ashu Dutt
Stop Losing Start Winning

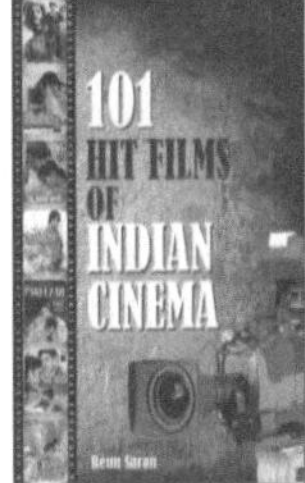

Renu Saran
101 Hit Films of Indian Cinema

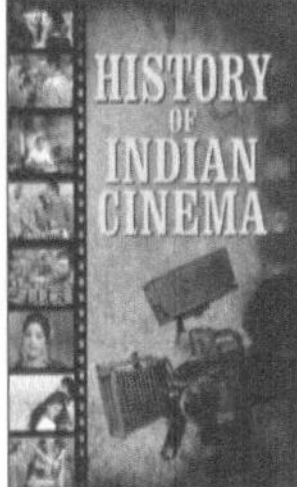

Renu Saran
History of Indian Cinema

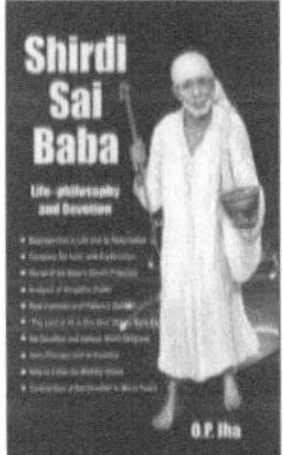

O.P. Jha
Shirdi Sai Baba: Life Philosophy and Devotion

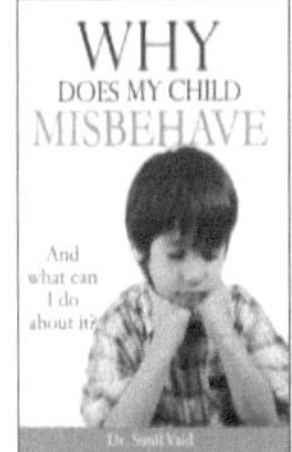

Dr. Sunil Vaid
Why Does My Child Misbehave

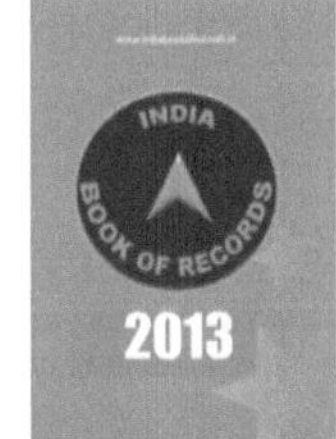

Biswaroop Roy Chowdhury
India Book of Records

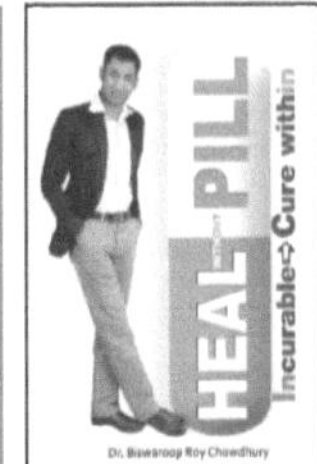

Biswaroop Roy Chowdhury
Heal Without Pill

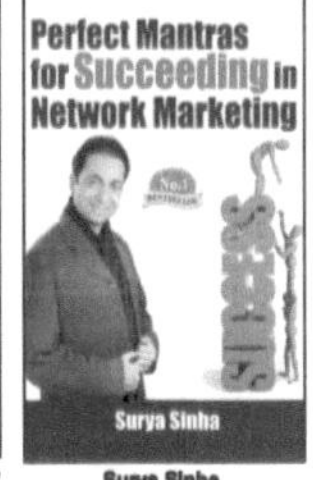

Surya Sinha
Perfect Mantras For Succeeding in Network Marketing

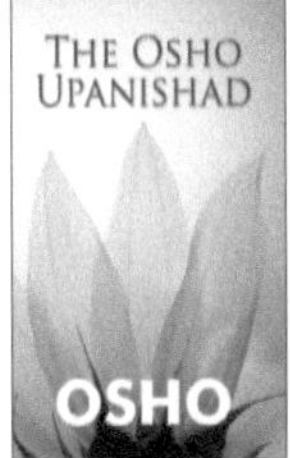

OSHO
The Osho Upanishad

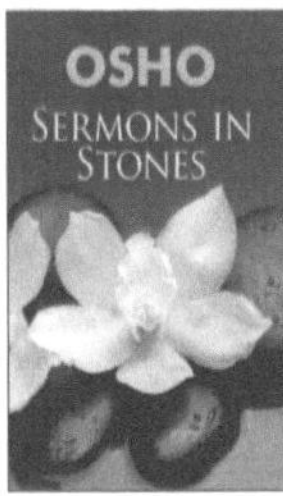

OSHO
Sermons in Stones

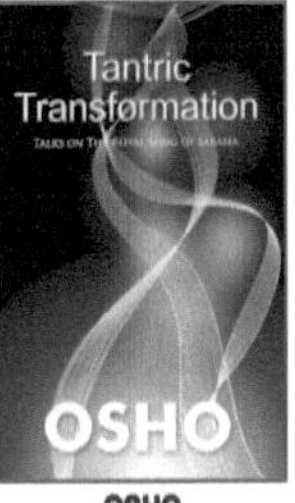

OSHO
Tantric Transformation

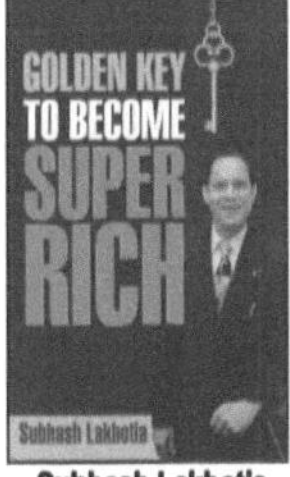

Subhash Lakhotia
Golden Key to Become Super Rich

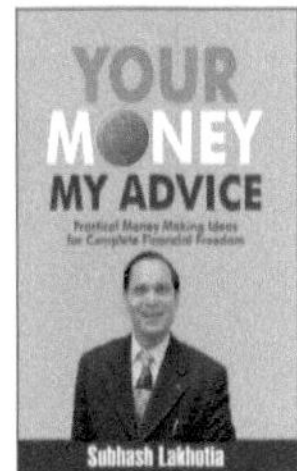

Subhash Lakhotia
Your Money My Advice

DIAMOND BOOKS X-30, Okhla Industrial Area, Phase-II New Delhi-110020
Tel : 011-40712200 email : sales@dpb.in
Shop online at www.diamondbook.in

www.ingramcontent.com/pod-product-compliance
Ingram Content Group UK Ltd.
Pitfield, Milton Keynes, MK11 3LW, UK
UKHW041827200726
13854UKWH00002BA/644

9 788171 825325